The
Survivor's
Mindset

kick-start your health
with the power of your
mind & body

BERNADETTE BOHAN

Newleaf

Gill & Macmillan
Hume Avenue, Park West
Dublin 12
with associated companies
throughout the world
www.gillmacmillan.ie

ISBN: 978 07171 5017 5

Print origination by Carole Lynch
Printed by ScandBook AB, Sweden

This book is typeset in Adobe Garamond 12pt.

The paper used in this book comes from the wood
pulp of managed forests. For every tree felled, at least
one tree is planted, thereby renewing natural resources.

A catalogue record for this book is available
from the British Library.

5 4 3 2 1

Dedication

To Ger, Richard, Sarah and Julie,
whom I love with all my heart

Note from the publisher

The information given in this book is not intended to
be taken as a replacement for medical advice.
Any person with a condition requiring medical attention
should consult a qualified medical practitioner or therapist.

Contents

Acknowledgements

My sincere appreciation to my dear friends Deidre and Geraldine whose love, support and encouragement I so appreciate.

To Michael Gill for his invaluable experience and expertise.

To Wanda Carter for her vision and common sense advise.

To the doctors who passed on their knowledge and guidance: Dr Brian Clement, Dr Felipe Reitz, Dr Udo Erasmus, Dr Andy Bernay-Roman, Dr Anthony Chatham and Drs Alma and Denis Prone.

To Professor Jane Plant who is an inspiration to those newly diagnosed.

To Orna, Agnes, Finn, Kathryn, Eileen, Jacqueline, Anne and Peter.

Last, but not least, for the immense contribution of those who have shared their stories so that others might benefit.

BERNADETTE BOHAN
FEBRUARY 2011

Foreword

Bernadette Bohan's *The Survivor's Mindset* establishes a detailed map of how someone can bring about their own recovery and renewal. When I first met Bernadette she was a frightened yet determined young woman after a conference in Dublin, she impressed me as a determined student of truth. Faced with the return of cancer, she launched her own one-woman, healthcare regime, and brought about her own complete recovery. Although this accomplishment eludes most, she has achieved her goal. However, as a maternal and caring woman, she could not return to the fabric of her rich and fulfilling life as wife and mother without enlarging her sphere of influence.

Writing her first book that reflected practical procedures much like a detailed diary, she was elevated internationally to a privileged position as a spokeswoman for common sense approaches to treating cancer. Being able to observe and know her over this transformative period gave me the privileged insight to experience an emerging force. Bernadette's confidence grew as she set out on a higher road to help more of the suffering masses. Her initial reluctance to speak to individuals and groups about her transformation fell to the wayside as the calendar rolled on. Finally, there was enough time between her initial diagnosis and ultimate announcement of recovery to embrace the many textures and nuances that had become part of her persona.

Only a couple of years ago, we discussed her thoughts on survival and how central the mind and its potential focus are in creating this reality. She, just like thousands of others with whom I have worked here at Hippocrates, embraced the revelation that it is our imagination and actions that guide our future. Healing begins head first. Many prerequisite tools are required to finalise the act, such as diet, exercise, etc. Foremost is finding your purpose and pursuing its fulfilment relentlessly. Bernadette has become a master in this foundational process. She articulates on the pages of this book as well as the numerous conferences and seminars that she conducts, *truth* at its best. There is no greater teacher than one who has experienced control over their own destiny.

Once an enthusiastic student of mine, Bernadette has now become a colleague in the important work of renewing humanity's health and soul. She is a formidable force for those who are willing to face themselves and make the necessary changes that are required for recovery and survival. There are many philosophers who talk of what they have never experienced, and then there are a few who speak from their heart about their own renewal. It is time that all serious people, ill or well, prepare for a voyage into the natural world of comprehensive totality.

The Survivor's Mindset is a must-read for all standing on the edge of the figurative cliff. Tenuous fear mixed with extraordinary exhilaration portrays that awkward yet inspired place. After devouring the poignant words of this pure, simple and profound woman, you will be ready to spread your wings and fly freely into the endless potential that awaits.

DR BRIAN CLEMENT
HIPPOCRATES HEALTH INSTITUTE

Chapter One

The Big 'C'

'A man must make his opportunity, as oft as find it.'

FRANCIS BACON

It was official, it was real, it was happening again. I had cancer – the big 'C'. I couldn't believe it, my heart pounded in my chest, the colour drained from my face and my stomach began to do somersaults as my doctor confirmed the results of the mammogram. The stomach-lurching experience of becoming a cancer patient again – or worse a cancer victim facing the terrifying possibility of dying before my children had grown up – was in stark contrast to my life as a happy mother.

The news was overwhelming, yet I knew I had to be strong. It may be a cliché but, from that moment on, it was my path. Now I really had to wise up if I was to reshape the life that I so desperately wanted to hold on to. What a painful way to learn the value of health. If only I had listened to my natural instincts and a little common sense earlier, I might have had the foresight to take care of my health and prevent this desperate situation arising. But, of course, it's easy to be wise with hindsight. With so much going on in the house with my young children, the everyday dramas of family life had taken over my daily routine – as it does for most mothers.

Twelve years earlier, when I was 33 years of age, married with two small children, I had developed cancer of the lymph system. Pregnant at the time, the shock of the diagnosis led to me losing my baby. I was advised by my doctors not to have any more children as it might have been the pregnancy hormones that triggered the cancer. At that stage, I took the medical advice and treatment, and did as I was told. I went home with armfuls of drugs and felt completely helpless.

After living for seven years free of cancer, I believed I'd been cured. Driven by a compulsion stronger than sense, I made the choice to have another baby. I knew that it could work out to be a reckless decision, but the longing for another child was so deep and instinctive that I decided to take that chance. After all, life is for living and where would we be in life if we never took any risks? My selfish, reckless decision brought no rush of congratulations from my doctors, who had been telling me for many years to put the thought of another child out of my mind. Thankfully for us, this was one piece of advice I didn't listen to and the decision turned out to be a blessing. Our third child, Julie, the joy of our lives, was born safe and sound.

The Frightened Patient

Five years after Julie had been born, and having been told that I had cancer again, I could not believe that I found myself back in the same place I'd been 12 years earlier. It was my lowest point, but

I picked myself up and decided I would not let circumstances take over. Whatever the outcome was going to be, I was not about to sit on the sidelines and wait until I got to the point of no return. I had to find a way to help myself.

I began to wonder if there was something – anything – I could do to improve my situation. I felt that I had to take some personal responsibility for my health – I couldn't leave it all to the doctors. When diagnosed with a life-threatening disease, you soon learn to focus. I decided to go with my first instinct and see if what I was eating and drinking would make a difference.

I set about examining the fundamental role of nutrition and diet. Surely it was worth a try? I was excited and fearful at the same time but I had to start somewhere, I couldn't mope around and do nothing. I had to embrace any changes with open arms if I was to bring about a disease-free future. Nothing would dampen my enthusiasm, I would channel all my energy into becoming informed on health. Time was valuable and the sooner I got on with the job, the greater my chance of success.

I am a very pragmatic person and it seemed to me that there might be things I could do that would not only help me through the operation, chemotherapy and radiation I was facing, but that would also help me to recover from the cancer itself. With these new thoughts, I became determined to save my life. My mother's words – 'Where there is a will, there is a way' – had a new meaning for me now.

I definitely inherited my first interests in health from my mother. Decades ago, parents passed on to their children the valuable lessons of healing they had learned from their own mothers and fathers. Many of these practices go back to antiquity and were handed down carefully. Such knowledge was commonplace in my childhood and it greatly benefited everyone. Despite having no formal medical training, people recognised the value of that wisdom.

My own mother, who lived to the ripe old age of 93, recognised nature's wonderful self-healing mechanisms perfectly too. She had a special appreciation of this disappearing knowledge, yet she had never read a health book in her life. She seemed to have an instinctive understanding of the fundamental principles of health, and managed to raise a family of seven through life's ups and downs. I vividly remember how, when we were children, she would 'doctor' us when we were sick. I remember being put to bed with warm drinks, no food and given plenty of rest – and I stayed in bed until the colour came back to my cheeks. No matter how long it took, she would not allow me to return to school until I was fully recovered.

This was her instinctive remedy for a child who was poorly. She recognised perfectly nature's combined needs for rest and liquids. Unfortunately, in today's fast-paced world, few people are given time to recuperate in this natural way. The healing process of nature is speeded up or taken over by medicines, such as antibiotics and anti-inflammatories. Sadly, the hectic pace of our modern world means that few of us have the time it takes to heal at nature's pace.

Looking back to my youth in a small Irish town, there were most definitely no visits to the doctor for antibiotics. My mother never bought into the idea of relying on doctors – partly because of her own instinctive wisdom; partly because she was not indoctrinated, as so many are today, with the idea that conventional medical care is the only valid way; and, to be honest, I think also because she had little money to lavish on such visits. I recognise now that my mother treated ailments of every description as competently as any medical person.

But times have changed dramatically and, today, we depend on the latest ground-breaking discoveries of modern medicine to *fix* us. We are all too ready to dash to the GP at the first twinge or sniffle and delegate responsibility for our well-being to our doctors. Maybe it's because, that way, if they make the decisions for us and get it wrong, we have someone to blame. I believe we no longer trust ourselves when it comes to healing and this is a loss that is costing us dearly in terms of health and well-being.

My mother was definitely instrumental in teaching me that it is natural for the body to heal itself. In retrospect, I wonder if I would be so open minded to nature's healing in my life today, if she had not demonstrated the importance of recognising the ability each of us has to heal. Her open-minded teaching was a blessing and it freed me to follow new approaches.

Because my mother had given me such a strong sense that I was responsible for my own healing, the second time I was diagnosed with cancer, I decided to check out if natural remedies were as relevant today as they had been in my childhood. I was desperate for information that would provide some sort of solution to my dilemma – without it, I felt at a serious disadvantage.

As I have a strong belief that understanding and knowledge give you control, I began to educate myself on the subject. I wanted to find out how to treat the cause of my disease and not just the symptoms. Maybe in the annals of nutritional health, there was information that could make a difference to someone with cancer.

Even having had such a marvellous example of personal responsibility and intuitive natural healing, up to that point in my life, health had remained a passing interest for me, limited to occasionally reading a health book or article in a magazine. I felt naively secure in the knowledge that I was leading a fairly healthy life. I realise now that I had learned little from the first time I had developed cancer – but this time, desperation led me to that much-needed education and I learned the importance of it the hard way.

Despite my inner conviction that I was doing the right thing, everyone around me seemed to think I was clutching at straws. I was driven by curiosity. This second cancer diagnosis made me realise that I really had to step up to the mark, bite the bullet and take responsibility for my health and well-being. My mother's healing abilities were at the forefront of my mind. She had a toughness and inner resilience about her, and I would need that same quality more than I could ever have imagined. I asked myself what she would have done in my situation and the answer came – she would have rolled up her sleeves, mustered up whatever weapons were available to her and followed it right through to the end.

This had been the key to her success and, now, I felt my life depended on tapping into these skills. I decided I would follow in her footsteps and try to learn everything I possibly could to help myself. The time had come for me to claim back my health and give myself a future.

The Desperate Student

Looking back, I realise that I'd thought I was fairly up to date on health matters. How wrong I was.

I had some health books on the shelf in my bedroom, so I started with them. As the one thing I could do was read, I read from that point onwards as if my life depended on it. I read selectively at first, avoiding books on chemotherapy and radiation because I was not yet ready to know about the gory details of those treatments, which I had not had to face the first time I'd had cancer. I took it one step at a time, absorbing what I could.

I started to find out about lectures and talks, and I began to make notes; the notes became a file and the file became a library. The mass of information I was accumulating was in some ways mind-boggling but, in other ways, mind-expanding, but my need to understand what was happening to me and what I could do about it kept me going. Locating information on how to optimise my chances for health and recovery was easy, yet so much of it was conflicting. There appeared to be no clear-cut answers. How could I cut through the maze of information? I began to wonder if this *was* rocket science. Still, I collected the conflicting data and continued to read and read, determined to find answers.

Some of the questions that ran in circles around my mind were: Is our physical well-being dependant on the food we eat? If so, then why does conventional medicine avoid the whole area of diet and nutrition in the treatment of cancer? Is poor diet a factor in creating a vulnerable immune system that enables cancer to develop?

It was at this stage that I stumbled across a copy of *The China Study*. As I lifted it from the shelf in the bookshop, I knew it was a book I had to read. The study pointed out the most powerful weapon against diseases such as cancer is the food we eat every day. I read on: 'Change your diet and dramatically reduce your risk of cancer.' Suddenly, I felt clear-headed and positive – this was the information I'd been looking for.

The study was recognised by *The New York Times* as the 'largest most comprehensive study ever undertaken on the relationship between diet and disease'. *The China Study* was the culmination of a 20-year partnership between Cornell University, Oxford University and the Chinese Academy of Preventive Medicine. In it, the author, Dr Colin Campbell, detailed the connection between nutrition and heart disease, diabetes and cancer, and the ability of the foods we eat to reduce or reverse the risks or effects of these deadly illnesses.

At the outset of his research, Campbell explained how he never could have guessed that food was so closely related to health problems. He began with an in-depth study into protein and the causes of cancer. He found that the people who ate the most plant-based foods were the healthiest and tended to avoid chronic disease and that the people who ate the most animal-based foods suffered more with chronic diseases. His findings also suggested that when a potent carcinogen (cancer-causing substance) is put into the body, the rate at which it causes problems is mostly controlled by nutrition.

The study had examined 6,500 adults in more than 2,500 counties across China and Taiwan, and produced more than 8,000 statistically significant associations between dietary factors and disease. Dr Campbell concluded that: 'These results could not be ignored.' *The China Study* has been described as the definitive study on diet and nutrition and conclusively demonstrates the link between nutrition and heart disease, diabetes and cancer.

The evidence of this monumental survey led me to continue my research and I found further evidence from the Bristol Cancer Centre's database that clearly pointed to the connection between diet and cancer. The World Cancer Research Fund also states that a high plant-based diet may reduce the incidence of cancer. I remember thinking to myself, 'If only I had learned all of this information earlier in my life! Why had I waited till my choice was so desperate?' The implication that it was down to breakfast, lunch and dinner made me realise I had to try this out for myself.

It appeared that the only option available to me where I could make a difference was what went into my shopping basket. And I didn't want to waste time wondering if it was the environment or some other unknown that had given me cancer.

What really puzzled me was that if it was true that nutrition plays such a big part in combating the effects of degenerative diseases that affect so many of us in the Western world, why wasn't more money being spent on this type of research? Many cancer sufferers ask me why, if the research indicates that diet can be such an effective tool against cancer alongside standard medical interventions, is it ignored in their treatment programmes?

I remember that I found it very frustrating and disappointing at the time to discover that none of my doctors was able to give me definite answers about why I had developed this disease for a second time – or, indeed, why I had developed it in the first place!

The scientific results of all the studies I was reading may have been convincing but I found those in opposition to them directed a wave of cynicism towards the research belittling the value of some of the new evidence. Unfortunately, in many fields of science and medicine, a great deal of effort goes into cataloguing why something will *not* work. As the theoretical aspects and practical applications are being sorted out, we the patients end up with a confusing minefield of contradictions that needs further clarification.

While I agree an objective opinion is valuable, it's like everything else when you enter a shadowy, grey area – it is susceptible to multiple interpretations. Patients end up waiting for further scientific evidence to prove the new findings beyond a shadow of a doubt, but some of us cannot afford to sit around and wait until there is conclusive, scientific proof. Scientific proof is of little value to the person facing the ravages of a deadly disease such as cancer, they must start somewhere to turn their lives around, regardless of the scientific evidence.

I needed a solution I could employ straightaway, not at the end of a two-year double blind trial. But there was no point in having a survival strategy that would neglect the basic principle of healing, that made no sense to me. I decided to trust Mother Nature and use nothing but fresh, raw, unprocessed foods – the finest medicine that nature can provide. A regular supply of food that is not stripped of its immune-boosting nutrients would provide me with the best essential components for health and recovery. The research showed that it is imperative to provide your body with food that has immune-boosting nutrients, enzymes, probiotics and antioxidants in order to help it recover and thrive. The extraordinary mechanisms of living foods promote immunity and have the ability to protect our cells.

As actions speak louder than words, I knew it was not enough to just collect the information, I had to be prepared to put it into practice. I always feel better when I am doing something, so I made a to-do list to help me get started. I began juicing and adding nourishing foods – such as alfalfa, fenugreek and broccoli – to my daily routine. I concentrated only on the foods that I could eat and, rather than resist temptation, I avoided it. I cleaned out my cupboards of anything I did not want to go into my body. This ensured that I would not be tempted and, somehow, I didn't feel deprived trying to resist biscuits, cheese and chocolate. I made a list of natural supplements to take and I also made sure that I took some time out to rest and relax. These proactive steps soon became ingrained into my daily life.

Initially, I realised that the chemotherapy and radiation treatments were going to be very debilitating and I worked hard to try to counteract the effects on my immune system. What happened next amazed me! I had never experienced healing to this extent on a physical level before. As I switched to more nourishing foods, I first began to notice the disappearance of the arthritis in my right hand and shoulder that had plagued me for many years. This was a significant turning point for me as I could feel the benefits happening. I'd worn reading glasses since I was 16, but realised that I was picking them up less and less. My bleeding gums vanished and the pain in my lower back that I attributed to lifting my daughter Julie subsided. As an added bonus, I also lost my middle-aged spread!

I welcomed these positive secondary gains with open arms, but having arthritis and wearing reading glasses are not such major problems when you have been diagnosed with cancer. I was looking at the bigger picture. I was hoping to heal myself from cancer and the side effects of its treatments. Of course, I couldn't see the cancer itself, but I could see these welcome changes to my body. This positive feedback from my body was confirmation to me that when you give your body what it needs, it will speed recovery and reward you by supporting the natural state of health.

I realised then that by boosting the immune system I had put my body *back in charge.*

Encouraged by the positive changes that were happening to my body, I became more and more confident that nutrition was the bottom line when it comes to good health. Now it seemed a logical and a natural step to investigate how to make tasty meals that my whole family could eat. After all, how difficult could it be to switch to foods which, according to what I was reading, could help me fight this disease?

Sometimes, we automatically assume that eating healthy food will be tasteless and awful. One reason for this is possibly because we don't know how to prepare and combine nutritious foods in an appetising way. This was another area where I was keen to learn more. So I taught myself to prepare healing juices, scrumptious salads, snacks, dips, mouth-watering main meals and yummy, nutritious, guilt-free treats with almonds and raisins to add a little sweetness to my life. All of them packed with nutrients.

My next bit of reading was about the importance of water – but I found it quite disturbing to read about the dangers of drinking tap and bottled water in Ireland. While I knew about the import-ance of drinking water regularly and that a sufficient quantity of clean water is necessary to keep the body healthy, I was unaware of the chemical cocktail that the average water supply contains. I was appalled when I discovered that substantial evidence exists that linked prostate, colon and rectal cancers to chlorinated water. The chlorine that is added to the water supply in order to kill germs is also used for fumigating, bleaching and disinfecting.

Fluoride is another chemical that is used extensively. The chief chemist from the US National Cancer Institute, Dr Dean Burk, began a crusade against fluoridating public water supplies when he conducted large epidemiological studies into fluoridated water. Burk concluded that adding fluoride to drinking water was an utter catastrophe for public health.

Barry Groves wrote in his book, *Fluoride: Drinking Ourselves to Death*:

> *Fluoride is more toxic than lead and only slightly less toxic than arsenic, yet it is routinely added to the drinking water of millions of people. They are given no choice. This mass medication is justified for reasons of dental health but there is no scientific evidence to prove the benefits of fluoride. Indeed all the evidence points incontrovertibly to the harm caused by fluoride to human, plant and animal life.*

The United States Food and Drugs Administration has clearly identified fluoride's toxicity by placing a warning on toothpaste labels and, to date, the fluoridation of water has been rejected and banned by 23 EU member states. That a poisonous insecticide, commonly used in rat poison formulations, is added to our drinking water made me realise I needed to clean the water coming into the house.

I checked out bottled water and found that this would not provide the answer to the problem. I may as well be pouring my money down the drain because the soft plastic bottles in which the water is often sold can leach foreign oestrogens (xenoestrogens) and other substances into the water before we drink it. Xenoestrogens affect hormone metabolism and increase the risk of cancers such as prostate and breast cancer.

With the rapid growth in the sales of bottled water, this is one of the problems that more and more people are becoming exposed to. I felt rightly ripped-off when I became familiar with these facts and realised that anyone who was serious about their health would have to go to some lengths to ensure their drinking water was free of chemicals and xenoestrogens.

Another issue that raised its ugly head was the use of chemicals in our pretty, packaged toiletries. Finding out about the harmful ingredients that went into everyday products like toothpaste, shampoo, deodorant, moisturisers, baby wipes, body lotions and makeup, made me realise that I needed to make informed choices when it came to my personal-hygiene products. The long-term effects of many of the chemicals contained in the numerous products we massage into our skin, spray onto our armpits, scrub our teeth and gums with, and clean our babies with are unknown.

I had never given a moment's thought to the impact exposure to the cancer-causing ingredients in these everyday products had on my health. Now, I was constantly scrutinising and checking labels – not an easy process – and sometimes it was difficult to get to grips with incomprehensible ingredients lists, typed in the smallest possible print.

At first I was reassured by labels that claimed their products were 'natural', 'organic' or 'hypo-allergenic' – but I soon found out that this language was sometimes meaningless, untrustworthy, even misleading. It often masked the truth. If you believe that these terms could not be used if they were not true, then think again. For example, 'hypo-allergenic' simply means the manufacturer believes their product is 'less likely' to cause allergic reactions when compared with other products. Companies see such labels as an opportunity to make larger profits, as these products often command a higher price. I found a good rule of thumb is to ask questions and then ask more questions.

In this book, I will remind you again and again that where there are vested interests, responsibility for the consumer's health is not always on the agenda. Much of this information is underreported in the media. However, the World Wildlife Foundation is one organisation fighting to ensure the chemical industry is better regulated so that the worst of these chemicals are phased out or replaced with safer alternatives.

Although what I was learning painted a bleak picture of the products I had been using, I also learned that there were many safe alternatives available from health stores, online and from distributors (see the Resources section). In the end, I found it relatively simple to switch to safe personal-care toiletries; it was just a case of buying them elsewhere.

Having read, sifted through and digested a vast amount of information, I came up with a plan that I came, in time, to call 'The Choice Programme'. A health plan that changed – and I believe, saved – my life. It involves:

- Fresh juice
- A few key foods
- Clean water
- Safe chemical-free products

The Attentive Teacher

Throughout my gruelling and arduous cancer treatment, people told me how amazingly strong and courageous I was. But what they said could not have been farther from the truth. I felt I had none of these qualities. Faced with cancer, I had all the usual feelings of anger, disbelief and incredible fear.

But no matter how discouraging or difficult it was to face this punishing and trying time, I kept coming back to one thought: I could give up and let fate run its course or I could find the courage to get up and get on with it. Courage, of course, does not change a situation: it merely gives you the strength to keep going.

Determination, education and focus helped me develop *a survivor's mindset.*

By educating and informing myself, I found that the knowledge I had gained gave me the power to help myself, and then many others. I never set out to become a teacher – it just happened, as people began to hear the news of my recovery. The first lady I helped shocked me when she asked me if I would lay out my programme so she could follow it. I never thought of it in such concrete terms: it was just what I had been doing to aid my own recovery.

Unlike my previous brush with cancer where I wanted to put the whole experience behind me, after my second diagnosis, I wanted to offer hope and show other people that, in the midst of their suffering and fear, there could be a ray of light. That ray of light was the practical changes they could make to their lifestyles combined with health education.

Soon the demand for the programme had expanded to include people with all sorts of conditions, including arthritis, cancer, Crohn's disease, heart disease, ME, fibromylgia and irritable bowel syndrome, and then those who wanted to maintain their health and prevent disease. I realised I had no option but continue, what-ever the cost. And, yes, there was a cost, mostly for my family whose lives were often interrupted by those with more pressing needs, but they learned to adapt and appreciate the value of what I was doing even when it cut into family time.

I became surrounded by eager people asking questions and looking for more information.

'Should I take supplements?'

'What do you think about meat and fish?'

'Is dairy good for me or not?'

My initial reaction to all the questions and attention was one of apprehension, but I had done the research and was practising it myself. The time had come to stand up and be counted and if I could help even one person that would be enough. Soon, spreading the word on the benefits of healthy living became my mission.

I never thought for one moment that I could stand up in front of an audience and deliver a seminar about all kinds of health topics. But when the opportunity came to get my simple message across at one of Ireland's largest health shows, I put my best foot forward.

I put together some notes on the benefits of my programme that I hoped would help others as much as it had helped me. Shaking with nerves, my legs trembling with anxiety and feeling the nausea that comes from too much adrenalin, I walked to the front of the room. Looking around at those men and women, I wondered what had motivated them to come. I was not an expert – just an ordinary woman, a mother. I was one of them.

I hoped my nervousness would not show. The room fell silent as I began to speak. I hoped they would understand the value of the four simple steps of my programme. Their need for more information on these subjects was palpable and I realised I was only beginning to scratch the surface. 'If I can do it, anyone can,' were my parting words on that day.

One woman from the audience – a nurse – came up to me and said, 'This makes perfect sense to me. I have learned more from you in one day than I have from all the guys with the PhDs.'

'It's just common sense,' I replied.

'Yes, but common sense is not all that common,' she said smiling.

A young man studying bio-chemistry congratulated me and a doctor from Galway asked my advice about grape-seed extract and blue-green algae. What had brought these professionals to my talk? Surely this information was nothing new to them? It must have been taught in medical school? I could not believe the response, it was massive and, in some ways, more than I could handle.

People wanted information packs, books, DVDs, juicers, water filters and sprouting kits. I explained that I did not have a business, that I was just passing on the steps I had taken to improve my health.

As I tentatively set about responding to people's queries, I knew I had captured their interest with my common-sense programme. I have now taught cancer patients (young and old), doctors, nurses, scientists and many other professionals about my prog-ramme, passing on details of the four steps that have helped me return to good health.

In recent years, I have also added another step to my programme when I discovered that so many problems originate from stress, negative emotions and trauma. Helping people address their mental limitations has opened up a whole new world of knowledge and friendship for me.

Over the years, I have become close to many people, some of whose stories you will read in this book. For every person that gets to write their biography, there are millions who never get to tell their stories. This is my attempt to tell the stories of Jenny, Martin, Laura, Amy and Maureen – ordinary people with ordinary stories that had extraordinary outcomes. For reasons of confidentially, I have changed their names.

I know from my own experience how hard it can be to see a way through all the information you are bombarded with from all sides – from friends and family, doctors, the internet and from your own reading. Simple, practical information is a lifeline for those people who are searching for a better way of living. This is not an alternative, impractical, flaky lifestyle I am teaching, just a wholesome way of dealing with all manner of issues that are part of human life.

In the same way that I had learned to live with cancer, accept it, and take what good I could from the experience, I knew I could help others do the same. I have to admit that I got a real buzz out of helping these people; seeing them return to better health was marvellous and gave me a tremendous sense of purpose. A good friend of mine, Grainne, who has been nursing for 22 years, says she gets exactly the same buzz when one of her patients leaves the hospital fit and healthy.

You can read my full story in my book, *The Choice*. It is the story of a very ordinary mother's life, but it is full of joy, heartache and tenderness and it reflects why and how so many people have come to listen to my simple message and approach, and why I believe nutrition and changing negative emotional states is the bottom line in maintaining good health.

What could have been the end for me turned out to be a new beginning. My past life as a frightened cancer patient and desperate student is a pale reflection of the life I now lead as a teacher determined to spread the word that nurturing your body with the correct fuel and building a survivor's mindset can make a significant contribution to your health. There are millions of people like me who are living proof of the positive effects of a better mental outlook and who advocate the benefits of nurturing your body with good food. You too can help your body become a picture of health.

Chapter Two

Real Stories, Real People

'*Often the hands will solve a mystery that the intellect has struggled with in vain.*'

CARL JUNG

The stories you will read in the following chapters are what have given me the motivation to write this book. They are just snippets from the countless number that came pouring forth after the publication of *The Choice* and *The Programme*, letters and emails from ordinary people – like you and me – who gained the power to turn their lives around, simply by being receptive to change. Even though they were dealing with life-threatening illnesses, they had refused to give in and, like a phoenix, each one of them rose up from the ashes.

I feel privileged to have touched the lives of so many people as we have evolved along similar paths. As we have communicated and identified with each other, we have found our paths were intertwined and often indistinguishable. We have had a genuine connection and I have found my true passion in helping the people who have sought direction, guidance and hope after they had received the harrowing news that they had cancer, or some other disease. Sharing our small and not so small triumphs, we have been bonded by our successes and failures.

As a token of my gratitude for my own health, I worked happily with them, in seminars or on a one-to-one basis, to help them remove any obstacles that stood in the way of their making the changes that were necessary to improve their individual situations.

When I asked for feedback from my readers, little did I realise the floodgates that this would open. The warmth of the contributions I received was amazing. I have used many of the letters and emails I received in this book – indeed, there were so many stories that those readers might as well have written this book themselves. This feedback opened a gateway into the lives of all these incredible people and gave me a first-hand glimpse at their achievements. Using this feedback as a starting point, I had the marvellous opportunity to research new and old methods of healing, and, in turn, this has helped me to bring hope and under-standing to those who need it most.

The feedback clearly indicated that mental attitude was one of the biggest difficulties people faced when they tried to change their poor eating habits and unhealthy lifestyles. There were many similarities amongst the different groups, and I found it easy to spot the downsides of making lifestyle changes for those who were stuck in their ways. This drove me on to investigate the pitfalls that they had encountered.

I have incorporated some of my own personal experiences in this book, too, which I hope will help you see that by eliminating unconstructive thoughts and feelings, it's possible to overcome stress, bad habits and emotional problems.

The motivating force behind The Programme was to provide people with a common-sense programme that would make it easier for them to implement the physical changes necessary to improve their health. In this book, I want to take this one step further and provide an insight into the mind–body connection and its inextricable link to our overall health. I am interested in finding real and meaningful ways to promote health and well-being.

As I began to learn more about the role the mind plays in healing, I felt it was incumbent on me to share this information with my readers.

The amazing power of the mind is an important component for health and healing and one that has been largely ignored and underestimated.

For many years, my home has been open to those seeking health and recovery. In the early years of my teaching, it was not un-common for my husband Ger to return home from work to find our kitchen packed with people wanting to learn about my health programme. The needs of these people taught me more than I could ever have expected. Thankfully, the majority of people I spoke to were in reasonable health, but there were also some who were not so fortunate.

In order to help these people, I had to find stepping stones that would enable them to get beyond the conditioning and limit-ations they had built up over the years. Apart from the practical steps about diet and exercise, I also told them about mind-control methods, such as regression therapy, counselling, hypnotherapy, visualisation, meditation, news fasting and journal writing – all of which are useful tools in helping people respond to lifestyle changes in a positive manner.

These methods offer mental and emotional support which help people stick to the steps of The Programme not just for a week or two, but for life. Feeling mentally and emotionally supported helped these people enormously as they began to step forward to reshape their future. As they navigated their way through their newly acquired information, they discovered they could use their minds to improve their health. This was a revelation for most, as many of them had been unaware of the role the mind plays in healing.

Although it is not possible to give an account of the benefits that every person has gained from following The Programme, I have, as I mentioned, received a mountain of feedback from people telling me about how it has helped them. I've had emails from Tasmania, letters from South Africa, and phone calls by the thousand from those who were closer to home. I have thoroughly enjoyed sharing in the accounts of these readers' achievements, some of which were outstanding. These people were genuine ambassadors for The Programme and I feel truly proud to have helped them accomplish such impressive results.

From the feedback I received from this wide and varied audience, I assembled a large collection of vital data which provided me with a tremendous source of knowledge about my readers. I found it very useful as it gave me a bird's-eye view of their success in sticking with The Programme, and also an inventory of the obstacles they had faced – and, I must say, there was a considerable mix of both. From this vantage point, three groups emerged from the responses. My natural curiosity then led me to broaden my research as I became intrigued with how and why people had similar traits when faced with the need to change their lifestyles.

The Enthusiasts

I named the first group 'the enthusiasts' because they exceeded my expectations in changing their lives for the better. They developed what I call *a survivor's attitude* – they had that determination to succeed that tells you straightaway that they will get it right. From the outset, this group appeared to be in control and had a talent for getting things done. They tended to be very task-focused, hands-on people who were determined to do everything in their power to succeed. They provided a good picture of the enormous success they had achieved. Many of those whom I met personally provided stunning proof that The Programme was effective; they were their own best advertisements.

Right from the beginning, they got stuck in and followed The Programme to the letter with many confirming that it instinctively felt right to them. Of course, they needed some direction, but they soon found the practical application of the changes laid out in The Programme easy to integrate into their lives. I recognised their enthusiasm and identified with how they were eager to share their experiences, feeling compelled to pass on to others what they had learned.

One of this group was a nurse who, in her spare time, volunteered at her local cancer support group to give reflexology treatments to patients of all ages and stages of the disease. It was amazing that she had spare time given that she was the mother of four young children. She had a huge interest in health and had first-hand experience of a group of women with breast cancer. She told me that these women carried out a daily regime of juicing fruits and vegetables and that she could not believe the difference this made in their appearance, energy levels and recovery rates compared to those who did not juice. She also believed that these practical changes inspired a turnaround in the mental, emotional and physical well-being of these breast cancer sufferers. She was so impressed with the results that she decided to try it out for herself. She wrote explaining that her juicer had been in overdrive since the group had introduced her to my book and she described how it was remarkable to notice the physical and emotional benefits that she was now also enjoying.

Beyond a shadow of a doubt, the physical improvements of this group was their best incentive, breaking away from their old habits gave them an understanding that it is they who are in direct control of their health. One change can often pave the way for another, especially when you begin to notice and enjoy the benefits it brings. Change creates its own momentum so when you put one success on top of another, you soon realise that every step makes a difference.

The Programme also opened up new paths for people in this group in many other ways. Conor, a taxi driver, was extremely pleased that the changes he introduced enabled him to return to his favourite sport, rugby.

As he had got older, Conor's lifestyle had become more sedentary, and, after a while, it caught up with him – he put on six stone in weight, most of it around his mid-section. Frustrated by the consequences of not eating correctly, Conor found he no longer had the stamina for the tough, demanding rugby matches he had enjoyed playing. He also had a very high blood pressure problem that his doctor had advised him to get under control.

Marriage, two young children and sitting in the car all day were the reasons for Conor's weight gain. Between fares, he snacked on chips, crisps and pastries loaded with trans-fats – and his big weakness, chocolate cake, did not help either. Conor laughed as he explained, 'I was getting so overweight, I was hardly able to get off the sofa. I really hadn't a clue about health. I suppose I was ill informed.'

His wife, Pamela, dragged him along to one of my seminars, hoping it would inspire him to lose some weight. Her plan worked and he became fired up to get himself back in shape.

'After that, we switched our focus towards whole foods, we ate more veggies and I took those omega oils. As soon as I began to feel a bit better, I promised myself I would return to rugby. I did this by picturing myself on the field, this helped me stay focused. It was especially helpful during the first six weeks, they really were the hardest. When I was tempted or had a craving, I distracted myself and focused on something else immediately. As Oscar Wilde once said, "I can resist everything except temptation" – so I avoided it. I soon learned to stop going into places where they had chocolate cake 'to die for'. When you're in a health challenge situation, 'death by chocolate' does exactly what it says on the tin.'

Pamela knew she had to be strong when Conor was at his weakest. If he'd had a bad day and deviated from The Programme, she got him back on track as soon as possible. She was a great help. She began juicing and making regular smoothies for the whole family and cleared out the fridge and cupboards of any processed or fattening foods. This meant that Conor was eating healthily by default because there was no treats or junk foods in the house for him to munch on.

She kept healthy treats on standby for his hunger cravings, these included nuts, seeds, dried fruit and popcorn. These may not be the purest treats in the world, but they stopped him eating junk food. Conor started losing weight almost immediately. Pamela helped him stay focused on his target and they celebrated his successes no matter how small. Eventually, he shed five stone.

'Once I got my head around the task, the intensity of the cravings started to lessen, maybe I was a bit more nourished. As regards eating out, I tried to make catching up with friends the main focus of an evening and not emphasise the food element in my head. I would offer to book the restaurant to make sure that I chose one where I would have a choice of healthy dishes.'

Encouraged by his huge weight loss, Conor returned to his long-held dream of playing rugby. He has continued to play, proclaiming that the rugby has kept him on track. Setting a target and staying focused on his goal helped him overcome his lack of energy and fatigue, it has given him a new lease of life.

As I sifted through the information gathered from this enthusiastic first group, I discovered that many of them had been spurred on by the fact that The Programme was genuinely easy to put into practice. Having on many other occasions been disappointed by diets that were difficult to maintain, they felt this programme helped them leave behind their old habits and move on.

Another surprising fact that emerged when I looked at the feedback from this group was how many elderly people it included. One of these ladies, Betty, was 86 years old when she decided she would take up juicing each day in order to help her painful rheumatism. Years of taking anti-inflammatory medicine had not improved the problem, and she thought she needed a bit of a rethink about her diet and reminded me that you are never too old to learn about and make changes.

So, contrary to the old saying you cannot teach an old dog new tricks, these people managed to throw off the habits of a lifetime. Experience had given them much more than grey hair, it had given them an understanding that change is not going to happen out of the blue. They had decided the time was right for them to make some simple lifestyle changes if they were to avoid the inexorable slide into dependency. More importantly, the time to begin was *right now*, they understood that the key step to any recovery programme is to start today.

How had these older people managed to be so much more successful than people half their age? Were they just the lucky ones? These questions helped me find the key to their success. I believe this can be explained in just one word: focus. My conclusion about these people is that the importance of maintaining their independence in their final years helped them stay focused on making a deliberate effort to take care of their health, as they felt they no longer had the luxury of time to take their health for granted.

The Dabblers

I called the second group that emerged from the feedback I received, 'the dabblers' because they had decided that they only needed to take on board those aspects of The Programme that already suited their lifestyles. They might have decided to implement a daily juicing regime, or clean the water coming into their home or buy fluoride-free toothpaste, but that was as far as they were prepared to go, for now. This, of course, is better than to do nothing at all – at least they'd made a start – but they didn't feel it was necessary to make the changes that would have made the big improvements to their health.

Essentially, most of these people knew they needed to make some changes to their lifestyle, because of the various health issues they faced, but they had convinced themselves that they were already living healthy lifestyles because they ate five pieces of fruit and vegetables and took a multivitamin each day, so they didn't think there was a need for too much change. They grabbed a few magic bullets but their old bad habits remained.

Angela was a perfect example of 'a dabbler'. She had had problems with reflux and had suffered with painful piles for some time, so she was clearly suffering from a digestive problem, which is easy to 'fix with digestive enzymes and proper hydration.

Indigestion and reflux are caused by too little acid or an inability to break down food. A simple remedy for it is to supplement your diet with digestive enzymes. Enzymes are small bio-chemical digesters that have the power to break down food. They liquefy vitamins, minerals, proteins, carbohydrates and fats to make it possible for them to be absorbed by the body. When we cook food, we destroy these enzymes. Even a partial reduction of availability of enzymes can slow the breakdown of food. Angela's painful piles were a sign of dehydration and constipation. Her colon was obviously finding it hard to eliminate and remove waste.

When I explained this to Angela, she was more than happy to take the digestive enzymes supplements but made endless excuses about how she found it difficult to drink water. She was prepared to do a bit to improve her health but it had to be easy and fit neatly into her existing lifestyle.

I asked Angela what she would like to change about herself, hoping this would help her to acknowledge that there was a need for her to change her approach to her health issues. Unfortunately, her answer was self-deceiving and she insisted that she was leading a healthy lifestyle. So she carried on eating the same foods that had caused her problems in the first place. At least the enzymes improved Angela's problem to a degree.

If we are to take advantage of what we already know about nutrition and health, we have to reorient our thinking. For many, it is necessary for them to change their existing thought patterns and belief systems in order to get results. This can be very difficult and, regrettably, some people cannot rid themselves of their old ways of thinking. We are more accustomed to sweeping these thoughts under the rug. For various reasons, we are all victims of the conditioning that we have absorbed like sponges throughout our lives.

On the other hand, if we allow ourselves to be free from judgment and to be open to new approaches, we can make the choice to change our negative patterns of behaviour. Only when we make a conscious and deliberate effort to look at our behavioural tendencies can we strip away the negative belief systems and behaviour patterns that have become entrenched in us over the years. A clear plan is important, otherwise you can so easily delude yourself. As your negative habits begin to fall away, it not only raises your awareness of your responsibility to yourself, it also empowers you to take control. I think of this group as a work in progress.

The Sceptics

Last but not least there was a third group that emerged from the feedback. The people in this group found it difficult to change their ways at all – and these are the ones to whom this book is principally aimed. The name I gave this group is 'the sceptics', because moving outside their comfort zone seemed to be virtually impossible. No matter how much they wanted a healthy, invigorated body, lasting energy levels or improved health, they still found it difficult to make the changes necessary.

At first, I couldn't quite put my finger on why this group struggled so much, but with some closer analysis, I discovered that a good percentage of them were inclined to be sceptical from the outset. For a variety of reasons, they could not see how they could move away from their old habits. Consequently, they were easily side-tracked.

They found it difficult to put into practice simple tasks, such as making juices or preparing proper food. They were 'too busy' and 'too tired' to fit these tasks into their lives. Of course the level of commitment differed from person to person but as some of these people were battling with serious disease, I was determined to find what obstacles they were putting in front of themselves.

I found nearly all the members of this group made instant judgments based on past disappointments. It is so easy to become trapped in a mindset of failure, but I believe we learn valuable lessons from failure. As Carl Jung said, 'Knowledge rests not upon truth alone, but upon error.'

This group generally started well and tried to make changes for about a week or two, but then, for a variety of reasons, they gave up. Before they knew it, they were back where they had started.

I was very sympathetic to the problems this group faced. I had made many mistakes when I first tried to eat more healthily and produced some awful meals as I tried to convert my family to a better diet. As you can imagine, this did not prove very popular and the experience did not help to persuade them that those foods were better for them.

But these problems should be seen as a normal part of the process of change, remember we learn to walk by falling. Thomas Edison made many attempts to invent an electric light bulb, and with each attempt he learned from his mistakes and turned his failures into opportunity. There is no such thing as perfection; we are all striving to do better. For me, the best way was to introduce the new foods one meal at a time and then, when that had become the norm, I would introduce another.

Another common denominator of the sceptics was that they did not get any support from their family and friends. Unfortunately, those who should have been supporting them, continually tried to convince them that the changes they were trying to make just weren't worth the effort. Although these people proclaimed to have their loved ones' best interests at heart, they tried to instil their own narrow views and limitations on the members of this group.

As humans, we are creatures of habit and so opening our minds to change is rarely easy. Familiarity is always viewed in an accepting mode; change is not. There will always be those who are ambivalent, sceptical and even hostile to change, in fact we often continue to do things just because that's the way they've always been done, and we don't question the old ways. The sceptics may not want to accept the facts because it puts too much responsibility on them to take control and do something to help themselves.

Conflict is the last thing someone trying to change needs as it is counter-productive, especially if they have built habits from which they have never strayed. We can't control how people behave, but it is possible to show them the way – even if they won't listen – by leading from the front. Your example may eventually influence the sceptics you meet. Experience has taught me that appealing to the taste buds of those who fall into this group is the best way to go.

Sadly, the sceptics were not willing to accept and experience personal change. One of these cases was Helen. Her husband Alan was trying to change his lifestyle but had been unsuccessful because he had found it difficult to convince Helen to get with the programme. The changes he was making even provoked disagreement with his friends, who appeared to be impartial judges. They called him a 'health nut', but Alan believed he needed to make some changes urgently, because he had no energy, his cholesterol levels were soaring and he had a blood pressure problem. His family and friends had an attitude of 'life's too short' whenever he mentioned the health and lifestyle changes that he wanted to make. It became apparent to Alan that although his wife and friends had good intentions, they did not want to move out of their comfort zones to support him fully.

This situation was familiar to me and I have seen it time and time again. If you take the example of a group of alcoholics, a person leaving the group presents a huge threat to his or her drinking buddies. It is so common for recovering alcoholics to experience hostility. I am afraid it's human nature to stifle the enthusiasm and efforts of others when we don't want our comfort zone to be disrupted.

I find it unwise to promise or preach the benefits of lifestyle changes to those who are not open to the ideas involved – it is something I normally steer away from. At this stage, I understand that the sceptics have little tolerance for subjects in which they have no interest. Most people are scared by change, and not everyone is ready for it. In fact, regarding change with scepticism and suspicion is very common. When we perceive change in this way, it is difficult for us to see clearly what the benefits can be. Perhaps if Alan's loved ones had had a better understanding and awareness, they might have been more co-operative and supportive and set aside their innate cynicism. Comedian Bill Cosby once said, 'I don't know the key to success, but the key to failure is trying to please everybody.'

Regrettably, for many of the sceptics I have met, having their efforts undermined led to poor results, and they achieved little of what they set out to accomplish. In most cases, I found that the impact of other people's views was the most important factor in their decision about whether or not to make the changes that were necessary – possibly because most of us define our successes or failures by the way other people relate to us. What a pity that they allowed others to stop their progress. If only they had been able to talk to those around them, they might have been able to explain the reasons they wanted to change their lifestyles.

When negative advice is aimed in your direction stick to your beliefs and follow them through. You make the decisions, bear in mind that it is your life and you are responsible for the results. You do not need the approval of others to change your situation (although I know it is helpful). Courage, conviction and commitment are all that are necessary – family and friends will follow eventually, even if it takes some time.

Alan's main problem was that he had never cooked or prepared food apart from throwing a sandwich together or sticking something into the microwave. He felt doomed to failure without the support of those who could teach him what to do. As he searched for a quick and painless way to improve his health, he asked my advice about to how he could make the changes he needed to make without this support. I asked him to come along to my three-day Wellness Programme, where I could show him how to cultivate a healthy lifestyle and learn to *keep it.* This course gave him vital access to information and demonstrations that helped him to implement the simple changes he needed. I also gave him a list of stepping stones to get him started and help him stay on track.

These 10 simple but effective steps have helped me and many others transform our lives for the better.

10 Stepping Stones for Changing your Lifestyle

1. Educate yourself

The essential ingredient for health is education. Our culture is studded with myths, misinformation and misconceptions about health and nutrition. If you are going to work towards a winning mindset, then you must develop your mind. Read or research the facts about health and nutrition and invest time in your health. It is the best investment you will ever make.

Good reading resources include: *Superior Health and Longevity* by Dr Brian Clement; *Cancer: Why we're still Dying to know the Truth* by Philip Day; *The China Study* by Dr Colin Campbell; and *Alive and Well* by Dr Philip Binzel. The impact of education is very important; otherwise health matters remain a mystery. When you understand the health improvements that come from making changes, you'll find it unappealing to return to living the way you used to live. Learn to ask the questions that you need answers to.

However, remember that researching in panic mode is not helpful, as fear dominates your thinking.

2. Make a pledge and declare it as a firm intention

Before you can make any changes, you have to want to make them. This is crucial – without being explicit in your declaration for change, you will have poor results.

Understanding the importance of the lifestyle changes you want to make is an absolute must if you are to respond to change in a beneficial way. If you want to succeed, the desire will keep you on track and help you to build a successful attitude. A proactive and positive attitude will put you in the driving seat. The more concentrated and focused you are, the fewer the doubts that will block your progress.

Be certain about what you want, your intention has to be defined clearly, otherwise your mind will be easily distracted. Distraction is not productive, remember if you don't have a clear intention, you only have a dream. Picture the outcome of the changes you're about to make often – for example, decide what you will do when you have excellent health. Are you going to take up a sport or visit a place you always wanted to travel to? It does not matter what your goal is, as long as it is important to you. If you have doubts about whether or not the changes will be worth it, remember that obstacles or challenges can either hold you back or make you more determined.

3. Set yourself targets

Targets will help you stay focused on your goal. They could include your cholesterol levels, weight or aerobic fitness, whatever makes it real for you. Picture the outcome as vividly as possible – see it, feel it, focus on it. You must have a vision and it must be at the heart of your every decision, it will help enormously especially during the first few weeks. This aspect is extremely important as these motivational pictures will help you realise your vision. A target will also help you to manage the daily tasks and keep you focused on making a deliberate effort to take care of your health. Above all, it will help you build a survivor's mindset.

Don't think too far ahead. Have a timescale for how long you will keep to The Programme. Plan to make the changes for a month, and, as the benefits multiply, you won't go back.

4. Surround yourself with *enthusiasts*

Make friends with like-minded people. It's a wonderful gift to share your experience with others and to see the positive effect you have on their lives. Finding others who will support your decisions and give impartial advice is a great help. This type of support can also free you from preconceived notions about health as you set about changing your ways. When you socialise with these people, healthy eating becomes the norm. The unifying force of these groups creates a wider understanding and enables you to speak openly.

Mixing with other health-conscious people can also prove to be the best possible way forward for you if your family are not really pulling together with you. Unless you have support, you're likely to be derailed.

5. Focus on the foods you *can* eat

How you think about food is very important. Concentrate only on the food that you can eat, rather than the foods you can't – this is the opposite approach to many diets. This simple tactic will change the way you eat for ever, because you are less likely to feel deprived of the foods you normally eat.

A change like this often paves the way for another change, especially when you begin to notice and enjoy the benefits it brings. Find healthy substitutes, there are a wide variety of products that you can exchange for your normal food choices. Some of these substitutes will equal or surpass the taste of the foods you have been used to eating. It is better to add good food to your diet, because a nourished body tends to have fewer cravings.

6. Make a start today

Make out a to-do list to help you start to make the changes you need – and do it today. Start juicing, add nourishing foods to your daily regime, and take some time out to rest and relax. Start slowly. Introduce new foods one meal at a time, especially if you are preparing meals for a family. Make one change and stick with that until it becomes ingrained into your daily routine.

Be consistent, because that way you won't be side-tracked and drift away from your goal. Without consistency it is difficult to succeed in transforming unhealthy and addictive eating habits.

7. Focus on what you *can* control

Don't get into disagreements with your family and friends. This is the last thing you want during a transition period as it will be counter-productive. Not everyone is ready for change and rarely can you control other people's behaviour. I can definitely vouch for that. Winning over their hearts (or should I say stomachs?) and minds can be difficult, especially if they are set in their ways. Instead of taking a firm stance and battling every day of the week with my children, I learned to develop some sneaky recipes – most of which I have included in my book *The Choice: The Programme* – and introduced new foods that way. If your friends and family are having problems supporting your new lifestyle, lead from the front, your example may eventually influence them.

When you are eating out, book restaurants where you can have a choice of tasty and healthy dishes and make meeting your friends the thing you are looking forward to most – rather than the food.

8. Supplement your diet with plant-based nutrients

Synthetic vitamins are not as effective or health-promoting in their isolated state as in their natural, whole food state. Certain herbs and plants contain antioxidants that have the ability to neutralise free radical damage in the body and also contain co-factors to protect our cells. The microscopic factors surrounding a vitamin are woven together in an incredible, masterful way. Even at the most basic level, vitamins and minerals will never perform fully without their co-factors, which, research has shown, maybe as nutritionally important as the vitamin itself. You get better results when you use supplements that contain all the co-factors to protect your cells. This is why isolated, man-made chemical supplements do not provide the nutrition that the body requires. We assume that synthetic molecules act in the same ways as natural ones, but many of them contain fillers and binders and are absorbed poorly by our bodies. Your body knows the difference, even though synthetic supplements are designed to try and trick it. Natural nutrients are absorbed readily because we are biologically programmed to recognise the naturally occurring compounds as genuine nutrients.

9. Remove the poisons from your life

As a society, we are ingesting pesticides, herbicides, synthetic hormones and growth stimulants through the food choices that we make. The result is that we end up with chemicals on our plates and there are health implications to eating this chemical cuisine. Nature provides us with everything that we need to live a healthy life.

You should also avoid drinking impure water by fitting a home drinking water system that will remove the contaminants found in tap water. Ninety-eight per cent of Western European countries have banned the fluoridation of their water supplies, citing serious medical and ethical concerns as the reason. Drinking water that comes in plastic bottles is not the answer as the plastic can contaminate the water with xenoestrogens (synthetic compounds that mimic the effects of natural oestrogens in the body).

Avoid personal-care products with harmful chemicals too – toothpaste, shampoos, deodorants, skin creams and even baby wipes have ingredients that can weaken your immune system.

Make sure that you look for organic products that are free from harmful chemicals.

10. Avoid, rather than resist temptation

Clean out your cupboards of anything that you do not want to eat. If you don't buy processed foods, you won't be tempted to eat them. When you are tempted or have cravings try to distract yourself and focus on something else immediately. If you have a bad day and deviate from The Programme don't beat yourself up about it; get back on track as soon as possible.

Do not go shopping when you are hungry. Hunger-fuelled shopping is disastrous. A little bit of planning is essential, otherwise you will be guided by your hunger pangs not your health, and you will end up buying anything and everything.

Using these simple stepping stones, you will ease your way forward and remove habits and beliefs that interfere with your ability to take control and change your lifestyle. They will also help you sustain change over a longer period of time. We all blow hot and cold when we are letting go of our unhealthy lifestyle choices, but sometimes change needs to be quite radical if you want to save your life.

Chapter Three

The Bigger Picture

∽

There is no question that the things we think have a tremendous effect upon our bodies. If we can change our thinking, the body frequently heals itself.

C. EVERETT KOOP, MD

Wouldn't it be nice if the human body came with an owner's manual or we had a definitive guide for surviving in the 21st century? We have specialists in every field with a multitude of different opinions and yet the average person has very little understanding of the basic mechanics of their mind and body.

Modern science is only beginning to understand the healing capacity of the mind. Recent technological and scientific breakthroughs in charting the mind–body connection have been astounding and we have now amassed incredible scientific evidence which helps us to understand the workings of the brain.

Evidence reveals that the brain contains 85 trillion cells, eight times more than the rest of the body and that this complex piece of machinery works 24/7 to maintain all the functions of the body and never shuts down – even during sleep. However, despite the increasing amount of scientific evidence, we have, as yet, had limited success in unravelling the mysteries and resources of the human mind.

When you begin to analyse the facts, you realise how extensive our brain evolution has been. Yet some experts believe we utilise only a small percentage of our brains, as little as 5–10 per cent of its total capacity. Surely if we could make use of a larger proportion of our brains' abilities, we could increase our intellectual performance. The following explanation at the workings of the brain has been simplified, but it can help you to see how we humans, special as we are, have not yet managed to access and utilise the functions of the entire brain.

The brain is described as the most complex organ in the universe, one neuron has 10,000 connections. Science has generated all manner of techniques to measure brain activity, but it cannot create a programme that has anything like the intellect of the human brain. Although this beautiful instrument of intelligence is far beyond scientific understanding, scientists at Harvard University are working to push forward the boundaries of knowledge. They are leading the way in terms of cognition and they have developed tests to measure what is termed 'the genius dip'. Their findings show that most children are born with extraordinary levels of intelligence – at the age of four years, 98 per cent of children were shown to have inherent genius qualities, but by the time they reached 20 years of age, only 10 per cent have retained these genius qualities, and, by the age of 30, this is down to only 2 per cent. The popular term 'use it or lose it' seems to have some relevance here.

If we start out in life being whole-brain thinkers, what is the leading factor contributing to this dip in genius abilities? Our educational system seems to have a bearing on this because it puts more emphasis on left-brain abilities, such as rational thinking, and cause and effect. Left-brain thinking is very important and helps us survive in our world, but constant left-brain thinking consolidates the neuro pathways of the brain and stifles our genius faculties, such as intuition, creativity and imagination. It appears that we all have genius qualities but they are often neglected or programmed out of us. These abilities may be lying dormant in your mind, and awakening or igniting the genius part of your brain depends very much on what you feed into your mind.

The Internal Computer

One way to think about the mind–brain–body connection is to view the brain as a 'biological computer', a control centre for receiving, interpreting and directing sensory information. The mind acts as the software that controls the brain, and the brain is the hardware that controls the body.

The content of the software is our thoughts. The quality of the software is important because our thoughts can be programmed with good or bad information. So we need to stop and think about what we feed into our minds. If we program our software with negative thoughts and behaviours, the brain will carry out the instructions it's been given. If the information is good, it may open you up to a life of inner strength, confidence and self-fulfilment; if it is negative, you are left to deal with all sorts of issues, including poor self-esteem, self-doubt and emotional insecurity.

Cell biologist, Bruce Lipton's research reveals how our learned perceptions control our behaviour and can even contribute to the rewriting of our genetic code. Dr Lipton demonstrates in his book *The Biology of Belief*, the enormous potential in becoming the master of your fate rather than the 'victim' of your programming.

We pay a lot of attention to our physical bodies but we also need to develop our minds and increase our awareness of negative thinking.

The brain appears to be more susceptible to negative thinking and it is the primitive, reptilian part of the brain that is responsible for this. Because of the reptilian brain's negative nature, it can be difficult to overcome the natural resistance to change it promotes. If you find you are constantly thinking negative thoughts, your internal computer may need a bit of an overhaul.

The first place to start when deleting negative programming is with your thoughts. The formula for effective programming and the key to success is focused thinking. The best way to do this is to focus on what you *do* want, rather than what you *don't* want. I found this useful when I changed to a healthier eating plan. I concentrated only on the foods that I could eat, rather the foods I could not. As my thoughts came into line with my actions, I didn't feel deprived of the foods I used to eat.

You need to be clear about what you want and then acknowledge that you are prepared to change. If you are working with a health issue, you must replace all negative self-statements, such as 'I can't' – your mantra has to be positive, 'I can'. One is empowering; the other is disempowering. Positive affirmations train your mind rather than allowing it to exist on automatic pilot. Your body will then act on these instructions. Henry Ford phrased this well when he said, 'If you believe you can or you can't, you're right.'

When you have clearly identified the benefits of altering your existing situation, you can discipline your thinking to accommodate your particular needs. The undisciplined mind is not in control, it analyses, procrastinates and gets very little done. When you have a crystal-clear intention in your mind, you can begin to change the nature of the habits you want to alter.

It is said that we are the programmers of our lives and life is the printout. If we underestimate the psychological aspect of our lives in a restrictive manner, we deny ourselves a valuable opportunity to progress and move forward. By ignoring the healing capacity of our minds, we cut ourselves off from a powerful source of healing. Remember a healthy mind together with a healthy body is twice as effective.

Silva's Mind Development Programme

My research brought me in a new and exciting direction when I gained vital knowledge about mind development programmes. The Silva Method was one of the programmes that helped me to develop a survivor's mindset. It was designed to give access to the full potential of the mind and encourage whole-brain thinking. This programme initiated many of the major mind-improvement programmes that are used today.

Many inspirational authors and speakers, such as Jack Canfield, Wayne Dyer and Shakti Gawain, have all tapped into Dr Jose

Silva's subjective education. Dr Brian Clement, director of the world-renowned Hippocrates Health Institute in Florida, explained to me how the Silva Programme profoundly changed his life. Having explored every approach and methodology before learning about the Silva Programme, he found that he was only vaguely touching on his potential. While exploring the ability of the subconscious mind, he discovered that, 'How we think, dictates our living experience.'

It took two decades of research for Silva to develop his self-empowerment programme. He had no formal education, and, in fact, the first time he went to school was to teach. Dr Silva wanted his children to have the opportunities in life that he had never had. He had originally developed the programme specifically to advance their performance in school. He had 10 children, and some were doing better in school than others. Silva found that reprogramming his children's minds improved their memories and increased their concentration and learning abilities.

He discovered that by relaxing the body and the mind, you facilitate what is called 'whole-brain thinking'. In other words, a deep, relaxed state gives access to the subconscious mind and enables you to use more of your mind. It increases your ability to affect your health, as well as positive life experiences and belief systems, and to access old programming, which may be blocking or interfering with your body's healing process. Dr Silva believed we are capable of solving problems of all kinds, regardless of whether they are rooted in the past, exist in the present or may even exist in the future. He devoted most of his adult life to this research.

Dr Silva devised a way for people to train their minds to overcome emotional insecurities, control pain, speed up healing, abandon unwanted habits and retrieve memories. His method is based on the fact that the human mind has multilevel states of consciousness. When we relax our mind and body, we enter the Alpha state. In this state of deep relaxation, we activate our body's natural healing abilities and are able to access the full potential of our minds to accelerate the healing process. This is one of the reasons why television advertising is so effective in promoting and selling products. When we relax and watch television, we enter the Alpha state. We are easily programmed at this level of consciousness which increases the advertiser's chances of capitalising on brainwashing us.

Entering levels of deep relaxation influences our biological system in a number of ways. Our brains receive more oxygen, cholesterol levels drop, cellular metabolism decreases, and physical tension and psychological stress are also reduced. Also by learning to use the power of your mind to change any limiting beliefs you may have, you can participate positively in your own healing process. In addition, these skills enable you to increase your ability to live in the present more effectively.

The development of these levels of consciousness helps you to pick up on stored information, release inhibiting and limiting thoughts, and grow your human potential. Using more of your mind and guiding it with Dr Silva's techniques, you can help to accelerate the development of a more positive, focused attitude, which is the key to regaining control not only of your mind but also of your health and your life.

The Techniques

The Silva workshops are designed to develop the creative powers of your mind and help you understand how your mind can be made to work for you. It also explains how to overcome the limitations of repression, irrational beliefs and negative emotions. The workshops are carried out throughout the year in most major cities around the world. The self-empowerment techniques for problem solving, sleep control, headache control and dream control are delivered over a three-day period. I have attended some of them and found that the techniques taught were surprisingly simple.

The process consists of a series of guided meditations or mind-directed exercises that steadily increase your ability to focus and expand your awareness of your internal senses.

The first stage of the programme is focused on teaching simple techniques to control and manage stress, and to become aware of your thought processes. The Silva Mind Development Method has been incorporated into the very successful Simonton Programme, which is discussed in more detail in Chapter 9.

Silva believed that by using the invisible, intangible part of the mind effectively, people can live a powerful life of their own design. A key element of programming your mind to become more focused is creating mental pictures at the Alpha level. This is because we retain 30 per cent of what we see and hear, 60 per cent of what we see hear and do, and 100 per cent of what see, hear, do and *repeat*. This is also the basis of the education system in most countries, where we use visual association with numbers and pictures to educate our children. The Silva Programme teaches people how to attract more of what they want into their living experiences and to develop the natural mental power of attraction. My own experience of this type of cognitive restructuring is that it certainly helped me boost my ability to retain information and tap into my creative side.

The ability to tap into the subconscious mind helps us in our struggle to control negative thoughts. Understanding how programming can affect our thoughts and behaviours could also help us change our habitual lifestyle patterns. Once we identify detrimental thought patterns, we can learn to replace them with beneficial ones. Imagine how tapping into the unused potential of your mind could enhance your self-healing powers, improve your ability to think and feel more positively, strengthen your motivations, and increase your compassion and empathy for others.

The inspiration behind Nintendo's *Brain Training* programme, Dr Ryuta Kawashima, shows that exercising your mind regularly helps improve learning and slows down the brain's ageing process. Over the past few years, millions of people are trying to improve their mental agility with these mind-training programmes.

Mind–Body Healing

Your mind and body need to work in harmony. Individually they have limited worth, but together they play an important role in the creation of both health and illness. Therefore we must pay attention to the impact of this interaction.

The World Health Organization's definition of health is 'a state of complete physical, mental and social well-being'. To put it another way, every part of the body is affected by the whole.

This two-way communication between mind and body is very real; it is not merely theoretical. What goes on in the mind determines what goes on in the physical body. For a very simple example of how the power of thought affects your physiology, close your eyes and imagine that you are sucking a lemon. Notice how your mouth begins to water. We have similar reactions to thoughts and emotions. When we get angry, our temperature rises, when we see someone yawning or scratching, it makes us react in the same way. These are physical responses to the information going into your mind.

A Fundamental Flaw in Treating Disease

Where did the notion that we could treat the physical body in isolation to the mind come from? Let's back up a bit and take a quick look at how the mechanistic way of treating disease came about.

The work of the 17th-century French philosopher and scientist René Descartes appears to be responsible. Descartes is known as the 'father of modern philosophy'. He argued that the mind and body were separate entities and he believed that the body could be treated in isolation from the mind. He did not believe in anything that could not be seen, touched or physically felt.

If we trace back the history of ideas to the time of Descartes' work, we can see how much of mainstream Western medicine is based on his mechanistic theories. His views had a major impact on psychology and medicine. Today, many scientists are challenging these views. Physics is an area where discoveries have led to conclusions that are challenging existing paradigms, and showing that a holistic approach is needed. Fritjof Capra is at the forefront of this revolution and he believes a new holistic, or integral, culture is on the rise.

Dr Capra's exploration of the paradigm shifts that have taken place in biology, medicine, psychology and economics have convinced him that we should abandon the mechanistic views of Descartes and take a more objective view. In his book *The Turning Point*, he says:

> *Before Descartes, most healers had addressed themselves to the interplay of body and soul, and had treated the patients within the context of social and spiritual environment. Descartes' philosophy changed this situation profoundly. His strict division between mind and body led physicians to concentrate on the body-machine, and neglect the psychological, social and environmental aspects of illness.*

While Descartes may have debated the validity of the role of the mind in physical healing, current scientific evidence makes it clear that healing does not only work on a physical level. Yet, despite the introduction of imaging techniques such as magnetic resonance imaging, that have given us a unique opportunity to peer into the brain, modern medicine continues to divide the mind from the body in the processes of health, illness and ageing.

Capra also wrote that:

> *The mainstream has become petrified by clinging to fixed ideas and rigid patterns of behaviour, creative minorities will appear on the scene and carry on the process of challenge-and-response.*

The dominant social institutions will refuse to hand over their leading roles to these new cultural forces, but they will inevitably go on to decline and disintegrate.

Dr Franz Alexander wrote in his book *Love, Medicine and Miracles*:

The fact that the mind rules the body is, in spite of its neglect by biology and medicine, the most fundamental fact which we know about the process of life.

Breaking through New Paradigms

The majority of us are guilty of paradigm blindness – we have sets of beliefs that we relate to without question and don't challenge. Whether they are right or wrong, they are often based on cultural beliefs that have become the benchmarks by which we live our lives. But life is not an exact science, even in quantum physics there are no definitives; there are, however, probabilities. Yet, we are continuously searching for scientific evidence to prove that what constitutes the status quo is the correct way to think. This is probably because change represents challenge, uncertainty and a denial of noble options.

New ideas are often ridiculed when they first appear, but we must realise how important the role of the mind is in creating health. Recent research in the field of neurobiology confirms that thoughts and emotions release encoded neuropeptides (short-chain amino acids) that help the neurons in our bodies to communicate. Recently many experts around the world have been working to increase public awareness of the benefits of these neuropeptides. The experts are not just a few dissonant voices, seeking to establish evidence of the role the mind plays in physical health, but pharmacologists, doctors and psychologists. Dr Candace Pert, author of *Molecules of Emotion* has conducted the most notable research. She has published over 250 scientific articles, discussing how a person's brain, glands and immune system are in constant communication through their emotions.

Her work on neuropeptides and their receptors can help us better understand the role of emotions and their effects throughout the body. Monocytes (key components of the immune system) have receptor sites for the neuropeptides, which link emotional responses in the brain directly to the immune system. It seems that our defence system is part of a complex network that links our intellect, emotions and body, and isn't just an independent physical guard against disease.

Pert concluded that emotions can change our body chemistry. She has contributed enormously to the shift in scientific research that is demonstrating how our emotions literally inform every cell in our bodies, including our immune system.

If science is showing that negative emotions influence the physical biology of illness and disease, letting go of negative feelings could not only be nourishment for your body, but could also be the start of a process that leads to the resolution of many other problems.

The Holistic Approach

Back in the 1940s, Abraham Maslow, one of the pioneers of humanistic psychology, also highlighted the importance of looking at the body in its entirety rather than as a collection of parts.

Humans are much more complex than a set of components. It is the person themselves who is the expert on themselves, rather than the scientist or the therapist.

While, for many people, this mental and emotional resource is largely untapped and remains something of a mystery, equally there are many well-accepted disciplines in every area of life that use the power of the mind for improvement. A good example of this is competitive sport. Lance R. Miller, an international shooting coach from the US, has said that:

Visualization, mental rehearsal, stress management and intuition are as much a part of an athlete's training regimen as diet, exercise, and sport specific practice.

Dr Denis Waitley has counselled winners in every field from top executives and NASA astronauts, to Olympic athletes and Superbowl champions. His studies with astronauts from the Apollo programme and with Olympic athletes, which he called 'visual motor rehearsal', showed what the athletes see in their minds is really what they believe will play out. He found that visualisation produced the same mental instructions as action. In the Olympic programme, he told athletes to run their event only in their mind. The same muscles fired in the same sequence when they were running the race in their minds as when they were running on the track. 'The mind can't distinguish whether you're really doing it or if it's just practice,' Waitley explained in *The Psychology of Winning.* Waitley concluded by saying, 'When you visualize, then you materialize.'

In his book *Healing Visualizations,* Dr Gerald Epstein describes the success his patients have had in overcoming physical illness by using mental imagery, including alleviating or eliminating rheumatoid arthritis, enlarged prostate, ovarian cyst, inflammatory breast carcinoma, skin rashes, haemorrhoids and conjunctivitis. He believes that image healing actually transfers the power away from the illness and gives it to the person.

He also recalls the case of a patient with carcinoma of the liver who had been told by his doctors that they didn't think he would survive, even with the chemotherapy treatments he had started. The patient decided to use visualisation techniques together with his chemotherapy for two years. After that time, he discontinued his chemotherapy treatment, but continued his visualisations. He is on record at the Memorial Sloan-Kettering Cancer Centre in New York as a survivor of this condition.

While many reports about the positive effects of visualisation are based on anecdotal evidence, it is worth noting that there are two major scientific journals devoted to imagery research: *Imagination, Cognition, and Personality* and *The Journal of Mental Imagery*. The information and insights recorded in these journals could not be more timely, since understanding all aspects of the ability of the human mind is crucial if we are to harness its healing power.

My wish is that people don't reject these ideas out of hand, these breakthroughs could change our thinking. At the end of the day, these findings and the developing theories based on them, will help us to increase our understanding and help us handle our emotions more effectively. This, in turn, could ultimately help us to live healthier, more self-directed lives.

The Placebo Effect

Another example of how powerful the link between mind and body can be is the well-known placebo effect. From the Latin word *placere* ('to please'), the placebo effect is a human response to the act of being treated, not to the treatment itself. It is the term used for a simulated medical intervention that can produce an improvement in a patient. The key to the placebo effect, whether it is the doctor's words or medical intervention with a sugar pill, is belief and expectation.

Although we do not have a biomedical understanding of how placebos work, they are a well-substantiated phenomenon that can have a profound effect on physical and mental health. The placebo effect demonstrates the importance of perception and the role of the mind in physical health. Research has shown placebos to be effective in reducing pain, lowering blood pressure, and, in some cases, apparently causing what is known as spontaneous remission of a life-threatening disease. Instances of the unexpected and inexplicable reversal of disease have been recorded all over the world.

Many physicians regard the placebo effect as a powerful tool in their armoury. In his book, *The Extra-Ordinary Healing Powers of Ordinary Things*, Larry Dossey suggests that:

> *All physicians should know that the placebo response is an indispensable part of modern medicine and a good physician must know how to maximise it.*

A good relationship between doctor and patient is vital in order to generate the placebo effect but, apart from that, the only other ingredient that is required is reinforcing the belief in a favourable outcome.

Henry Knowles Beecher was an influential figure in the development of medical ethics and research techniques. He was instrumental in the implementation of federal rules on human experimentation and informed consent in America. His seminal and influential 1955 paper, 'The Powerful Placebo', is still among the most frequently cited works in this area and is probably responsible for the double blind trials becoming a universal standard for medication evaluation studies.

His paper describes a study based at Harvard University that investigated the effects of post-operative pain. The first group of patients was given morphine; the second placebos. Fifty-two per cent of the morphine patients reported relief but 40 per cent from the placebo group also reported relief. If a placebo has the power to produce these types of results, surely it reveals how important our mental state is when it comes to treating disease. Ignoring this research will cut us off from developing ways to support the mind in its effort to treat disease. As Dr David Felten of the University of Rochester School of Medicine has said:

We can no longer pretend that the patient's perceptions don't matter. And we can't pretend that healing is something doctors do to a patient. Your mind is in every cell of your body. And your emotions are the bridge between the mental and the physical, or the physical and the mental. It's either way. Now there is overwhelming evidence that hormones and neurotransmitters can influence the activities of the immune system, and that products of the immune system can influence the brain.

The powerful role that the mind can play in the healing process may be difficult to take on board but evidence such as this cannot be dismissed. I advise people to evaluate for themselves, draw their own conclusions and to read more on the subject. There is a wealth of quantitative and qualitative data to support these findings and I've listed some of the most important in the Further Reading section at the end of this book.

Chapter Four

ASAP

'The beginning is the most important part of the work.'

PLATO

Two decades ago, the idea of treating cancer holistically was not even on the medical agenda. Today, there is a wider acceptance that an integrated approach can help us build not just physical strength, but also the mental ability to rebuild the body's defences. What I have found is that people are unaware that there are approaches other than the medical ones in the treatment of illness and disease. In this chapter, I want to highlight some of the other ways to tap into the brilliant resources of our immune system.

Mental management is paramount if we are to rectify damage to our physical bodies. Serious illness can help us see things in a very different light, though perhaps not at first. Indeed, during the initial period after diagnosis, we are very often overwhelmed by the frightening prospect of what lies ahead. Nevertheless, the body has a way of presenting us with what we fear most. While it may come as something of a shock at first, there is nothing 'chance' about disease. It is your body's way of attracting your attention, both physically and mentally, that you need to do something to help it. While this warning may stop you in your tracks, it can also be the spur you'll need to change your lifestyle sooner rather than later.

A few years ago, Jenny, a young mother, came to me asking for advice after she had been diagnosed with breast cancer. By the time she came to see me, she had already had an operation to remove her breast and lymph nodes and had undergone chemotherapy and radiotherapy treatments, she was also on a five-year treatment programme of medication to suppress her body's production of oestrogen.

Jenny had decided to make some dietary changes to help support herself during her forthcoming treatment. Looking back now, she will freely admit that, despite the diagnosis and the chemotherapy treatments that she was undergoing, she'd only dabbled in making changes to her lifestyle. When she had a recurrence of the cancer after 18 months, and had to go under the surgeon's knife for a second time, and undergo further rounds of chemotherapy and radiation treatments, Jenny tried once again to implement dietary changes in to her life, but many of her efforts were unsuccessful.

One cold October evening, she arrived on my doorstep in a daze, looking tired and strained. I welcomed her warmly, knowing from the look on her face that this was not a social visit. It was a day that Jenny will always remember, one much like the others that she had spent in her doctor's room having a routine check-up after some previous scans. In short bursts, she tried to explain to me how she had woken that morning with a lurching feeling in the pit of her stomach. She was anxious but, at the same time, confident that she was responding well to her treatment and that everything was going according to plan. Yet she had been uneasy as she set off for the hospital.

Her doctor was a kind, caring man with a reassuring manner, whom Jenny had come to trust. They often shared stories about their kids and holidays, and he was always ready to listen to her, even when she fired question after question at him. Jenny was hugely grateful to this man, seeing him as her saviour.

He looked up when she entered the surgery, seeming jumpy as she looked at him expectantly. He was shuffling his papers, his normal friendly approach somehow subdued and she felt that sinking in the pit of her stomach again. Nevertheless, she tried not to jump to conclusions, as she searched his face for information about the one thing that was on both their minds – the results of her scans. The tension in the room was palpable and he frowned as he picked up the file on his desk; he seemed too quiet and she noticed he did not meet her eyes. It felt totally different from her normal appointments. There was no friendly banter, no routine questions and answers, no chatting about the kids. Wordlessly, he motioned to her to lie on the couch.

She tried to read his mind, imagining that she could decipher her fate from the frown on his forehead and praying silently as he checked her all over. As the moment of truth arrived, she found herself holding her breath. He looked unbearably weary, but, somehow, he managed to maintain his professional dignity as he explained to her that the news was bad, the cancer had spread.

Her heart nearly stopped and she tried hard not to fall to pieces. She felt sick with fear.

'It's back!' she blurted out, as she walked into my kitchen. 'The cancer is back.'

She burst into tears, unable to take the strain of the worry and uncertainty any longer and allowing all her emotions to pour out. We talked for some time, during which she begged me for assurances that it would be all right. I understood only too well how frightening the prospect of the months of treatment that lay ahead was for this young mother.

'What the hell am I going to do? Jesus, I don't think I can go through this again, I don't know if I have the energy to fight it – the surgery, the treatment, blood tests scans and more scans. What if the treatment doesn't work?' she asked, searching my eyes for an explanation, convinced that I would have the answer. 'He said that the treatment would buy me time. It's not a cure. I have to find another way, as it looks like the conventional route is not going to cure me. It was bad enough losing a breast, every time I go swimming I am always trying to cover up rather than risk horrifying or embarrassing anyone. You feel like a freak when you've no hair. I know hair loss is minor and temporary – but I have just grown it back,' she raged on, through the tears that were stinging her eyes.

Jenny could not believe she was back in this situation, that history was repeating itself. The realisation of what lay ahead kicked in with her immediately. She asked herself why she had not seen it coming, but she had been a typical mother so absorbed in her non-stop family life that she had deliberately shut out these thoughts and carried on as usual.

A fleeting thought passed through my mind: why do mothers have such good instincts when it comes to rearing their children yet, they often fail to look after themselves? They are very intuitive at recognising the early signs of sickness in their children when every protective instinct in their body focuses on making their child better, a very typical – and very useful – attribute for a mother. I am fairly sure that if you look back at your childhood, you will remember your mother recognising that you were sick long before you knew it yourself, and Jenny was no different. She was totally committed to her family and her children always came first. This altruistic approach leads many women to forget they have an obligation to take care of themselves and not just their children.

After all the treatments Jenny had had after her first diagnosis and after everything she had been through, she had relished the distraction of a familiar routine of housework, preparing meals and walking to school with her children. Feeling that her children were more important, Jenny spent most of her time ensuring that their needs were met and learned not to expect too much for herself. Her concerns about cancer had slowly receded into the background of her busy life. But, like the predator it is, the cancer was merely biding its time.

As the awful truth started to sink in, she admitted she had always been a bit on edge about the possible return of the cancer. Some years earlier, when she had worked as a member of the cabin crew for a large airline, she remembered that the women had been asked to sign a statement during their training, so that they were aware that working in a pressurised cabin at 35,000 feet led to an increased risk of breast cancer. She contemplated the possible tie to her previous job and the cancer's return. Or, was it the contraceptive pill she had taken for several years prior to the birth of the children? She'd asked her doctor if that was the reason it had resurfaced. He'd said that cancer was difficult to categorise or find a cause for, he simply did not know.

As the tears began to well up in Jenny's eyes, I put my arms around her. She held on to me for dear life, needing me to be strong for her.

In many ways, her life mirrored my own. I can still remember the time I was first diagnosed, when my son Richard was seven and my daughter Sarah was only four years old. Looking at my beautiful children, I had to face the possibility that I might not live to see them grow up. I knew exactly how Jenny felt.

'I suppose I am only making excuses for myself, maybe I have been kidding myself that I was trying to make changes to my life. In reality I have actually tried to duck away from them,' Jenny said, as she paced up and down the kitchen.

I knew there was no point trying to persuade her gently into making the changes that had previously eluded her. If she wanted to get better, she needed to develop a survivor's mindset – and fast. I really needed to get across to Jenny that time was of the utmost importance. Sometimes to help a person work towards a healthy mindset, you have to build their knowledge and self-empowerment. The impact of education is very important, otherwise health matters remain a mystery. Education and empowerment would give control back to Jenny. I tried to encourage her to make a start and tackle things immediately. Obviously, my main reason for this was the urgency of her new diagnosis, but it is also the case that the sooner the body's well-being is reinstated after chemotherapy the better, as these treatments affect not only the cancer cells but also damage healthy cells in the liver, kidneys and other organs. The chemicals also wreak havoc with a person's immune system; some of them are so toxic that if they are spilled on naked skin, they cause burns.

Although the timeframe for disease progression varies from person to person, Jenny could not afford to waste valuable time. She needed to acknowledge that something had to change. She could no longer dabble with changing her lifestyle, she had to concentrate and focus if she wanted to get results. Her commitment was an absolute must if she was going to build a survivor's attitude.

Knowing that mixing with other health-conscious people could prove to be the best possible way forward for Jenny, I gave her details of an upcoming lecture. Explaining to Jenny once more that time was of the essence, I urged her to attend in the hope that the speaker's words would inspire her to make immediate changes to her lifestyle which would improve her chances of survival. She decided to follow my advice, took the details of the lecture and said she would attend.

Dr Brian Clement, director of the Hippocrates Health Institute in Florida and a leader in the field of mind–body medicine, was the doctor giving the lecture. The following day, I had a call from Jenny to let me know the outcome of the talk.

'How did it go?' I asked.

'I have made up my mind we are going to Florida, to Hippocrates. Everything Dr Clement said made sense to me. I am going to get stuck in and make the changes as soon as possible. Kevin [her husband] thinks I've gone mad, he thinks this is voodoo and pseudoscience, but he has agreed we will go.'

I sensed that Jenny had an enhanced feeling of control over her condition, but there was also urgency in her voice. She opted to travel to Florida with Kevin and the children to take part in the three-week programme provided at the healing centre.

The Hippocrates Institute was founded in Boston in 1957 and is based on the belief of Dr Ann Wigmore that the human body is a self-healing and self-rejuvenating organism if it is given the proper tools to function. Founded by her with Viktoras Kulvinskas, its goal is to assist people in taking responsibility for their lives. The institute offers a comprehensive programme of nutrition, complemented by mental and emotional support and appropriate physical activities – all essential elements for those on the path to optimum health. They also offer non-invasive therapies, such as hyperbaric oxygen chambers and far infrared therapy (there is more on these in Chapter 10).

Everyone who stays at the centre has the opportunity to detoxify his or her body and organs. This is a necessary step to relieve the immune system so that healthy cells can be regenerated, which, in turn, facilitates healing. There are eight elements to the programme which are incorporated to protect the cells from the synthetic chemical toxins to which we are exposed in our normal lives, many of which mimic oestrogens. This programme helps to purge the body of these synthetic hormones and toxic chemicals, to ensure good health and longevity, in the following ways:

- Far infrared saunas penetrate deep into the body tissues to release toxins, unlike conventional saunas.

- Hydrotherapy cleanses impacted waste from the large intestine. Cleansing the intestines periodically can ease the discomfort of a sluggish digestive tract.

- Exercise facilitates blood flow, keeps veins and arteries open and helps excrete toxins from the lungs and skin.

- Lymphatic drainage massage reduces congestion in the lymph glands and strengthens the immune system.

- Fasting with green juices and water is carried out once a week for a 24-hour period. This accelerates detoxification as it leeches chemicals from body fat. (They do not recommend fasting if you have blood sugar disorders or if you experience impairments that leave you weak.)

- Specific supplements of chlorella and blue-green algae help rid the body of heavy metals and the effects of radiation. Cayenne pepper, capsicum and garlic are also included.

- Rehydration with juices and water is vital. Water transports nutrients to the trillions of cells in our bodies, and it is essential in eliminating toxins and poisons and carrying oxygen to our blood stream. Our bodies are dependent on a regular supply of pure water.

- Wheatgrass juice cleanses the arteries and flushes out toxins. These juices protect against disease as they are rich in beneficial phytochemicals. Wheatgrass and its metabolic processes also assist bone marrow in generating new cells.

Ann Wigmore's lifestyle and research has contributed to saving the lives of thousands of people and Drs Brian and Anna Marie Clement, directors of the centre, conscientiously follow her teachings in a loving and supportive manner. Down through the years, the institute has seen a dramatic shift in people's attitudes to the role that diet and lifestyle play in promoting overall health. This shift in attitude has paved the way for more and more people to focus on attaining good health through psychological support, eating living enzyme-rich foods and availing of a host of therapeutic treatments.

As Jenny set off on the life-altering journey, I had great hopes that this young woman would find the help she desperately needed and also the commitment and determination to follow the programme provided for her. She was unlike some of the other people I had seen make this long journey. She was physically strong and did not appear to have been weakened by her previous treatments, although this was obviously just the outward sign; inside the cancer had now spread throughout her lymphatic system and had infiltrated both her lungs. During her three-week stay at the health centre, she found real practical help to implement their programme.

What fascinated Jenny was that many of the symptoms that she had associated with her illness were in fact her body's attempts to regain a state of health. Although this was outside her understanding of her disease at that point in her life, Jenny quickly rose to the challenge and embraced the programme fully. She learned about the wondrous ability of a properly nourished body and a healthy immune system. She learned how cleansing the body with green juices would assist her in helping her body to rid itself of toxins. This would help facilitate recovery and maintain her health while she continued the regime at home. I had some contact with her by email during her stay at the centre in Florida and I could tell that she had made a new commitment based on the knowledge she was gaining. What a relief that was!

At the Hippocrates Institute the daily routine for a patient like Jenny is to drink two 2-ounce wheatgrass juices and three 16-ounce green juices during the day, to eat a 100 per cent raw diet of enzyme-rich foods, have enemas and participate in an exercise programme for physical and mental well-being.

As I read Jenny's emails, I thought back over my relationship with her. Despite my sincere intentions to persuade her to take care of her health in the early months after her first diagnosis, Jenny had not been ready to change her lifestyle. On many occasions, I had tried, with little success, to get Jenny to stick to juicing once or twice a day. When I would broach the subject with her, she would laugh it off or dismiss it saying, 'I'll start again tomorrow.'

How had she finally found the commitment necessary to fulfil such a strict daily detox routine? It was simple; she was – quite literally – faced with life or death choices. The fear of the cancer killing her was greater to Jenny than the inconvenience of making these changes. Jenny had finally looked into the abyss and this had brought the clear focus that comes when one is faced with their own mortality. The education, skills and support offered at the institute gave Jenny the focus and determination she needed to change her ways.

On her return, I spoke to Jenny about why she had found it so difficult to change in the past and about her new-found commitment. As she contemplated what had brought about her change of mind, she explained with great honesty that she was so used to 'normal' food that she really didn't want to know the information, because she knew that if it made sense, she would have to take it on board. The practical side of dealing with her disease seemed overwhelming to Jenny, whereas the medical side was so well supported and catered for that she just left her recovery in the hands of her doctors.

Her new diagnosis had forced Jenny to look at her priorities. She has come to realise that true health must be earned, there are no magic pills or cures that can replace the natural healing of the immune system. The education had been an eye-opener for her. It changed her whole perception of her body's ability to heal and has been one of the key factors in removing her mental blocks which enabled Jenny to make the necessary lifestyle changes.

'Before my diagnosis I was feeling very tired and worn out, I suffered a lot with chest infections that I found hard to shift. Little did I know that dairy plays such a role in producing mucus. I used to drink a pint of milk a day and poured it into the kids thinking it was the perfect food for building strong bones.'

It was a delight to hear Jenny speak with such confidence and to know that the lessons she had learned would ensure she would avoid mistakes in the future. Jenny lowered her eyes as she explained how there were times when she had felt very alone going through her journey. But she had had the good fortune to find others at the centre who had first-hand experience of cancer who had made changes to their lives, Jenny found this very empowering. These people helped her to reaffirm her identity as a woman, not just a cancer patient. Jenny believes that nothing beats the under-standing you gain from experience and that the only people who can restore your confidence in these situations are the people who have travelled along the same road.

Jenny's new lifestyle has now become second nature to her and she no longer allows life's distractions to interfere with her ability to take care of herself.

'I have licked my wounds and I am ready to face the world again.' she said.

Her determination was clear.

Jenny's story once again highlights the mistaken notion that the physical body is separate from the mind in its struggle to achieve health. While illness presents enormous challenges physically, it also brings an awareness that mobilises us to change. It provides opportunity for personal growth that is otherwise not easily accessed, and it certainly brings clarity to the aspects of our lives that need it most. Those of us who have faced such a challenge can truly understand how a person's view of life can change. You have a new appreciation for life and it is even more precious because you came so close to losing it.

Gandhi's well-worn phrase, 'If I have the belief that I can do it, I shall surely acquire the capacity to do it, even if I may not have it at the beginning', certainly became a reality for Jenny.

To see her come through the other side of something as serious as stage four cancer is truly inspirational. Today, four years down the road, Jenny is in remission. She has clawed her way back to health and has now been given back the greatest gift of all – her future with her three beautiful children and husband. Her husband has also changed his sceptical mind, the three-week stay at Hippocrates Institute armed him with a new approach to his own health. He has applied the knowledge he gained at the centre and has introduced the dietary changes into his life with great ease. They are now totally committed to their daily routine of juicing, eating proper food and exercise.

This major challenge opened Jenny's mind and helped her to make herself available to the infinite healing within her own body. She is like a new woman, her vibrant looks paint a superb picture of the success of this courageous young mother. Jenny's infinite abilities for healing have now been unleashed and she continues to thrive. The moral of Jenny's story is start today, not tomorrow.

Chapter Five

Peace of Mind

'Imagination is everything. It is the preview of life's coming attractions.'

ALBERT EINSTEIN

My most serious experience of using my mind for healing came when I was dealing with the effects of chemotherapy. This was when I realised that finding a balance between mind and body was the catalyst for health and well-being.

Four months into my treatment, I had successfully managed to change most of my diet – I had cleaned the water coming into the house, I had thrown away the personal-hygiene products that had harmful chemicals in them and my daily juices were a lifestyle change I was very much enjoying. With hindsight, changing to a healthier diet had been relatively easy to achieve.

However, controlling my mind was proving to be a lot more of a challenge. To be perfectly honest, I felt I was falling apart psychologically. Although I was trying to remain positive, the seriousness of my situation was overwhelming. The loss of control and the psychological impact is difficult to explain: crushing feelings of fear, helplessness and hopelessness began to encompass every moment. On numerous occasions, I contemplated the possibility that the cancer would return; it was a constant worry.

When you have had cancer, you find yourself living with the possibility of its return every day of your life. Now my thoughts were filled with fear and anxiety. Keeping these negative emotions in check was presenting me with a real challenge.

I could not shake off the looming feeling of despair and uncertainty. I remember one night in particular when I hardly slept a wink, I lay awake worrying about the results of the tests from the operation; it was like living in a terrible limbo – a no-man's land. Although I was trying so hard to keep myself together and not overreact, a million worries passed through my mind: Would I live to see my little girl Julie grow up? Would I survive the onslaught of all the treatment? Would the treatment work? Would I end up back on the operating table having a second operation? All these thoughts, and worse, crowded into my restless dreams.

At the same time, I knew mine was a normal reaction. After all, I was no stranger to these feelings of anguish. I had lived through the psychological effects of cancer 12 years earlier – the first time I was diagnosed. The scars had faded, but the memories had not. While I understood that these were transient symptoms of fear, vulnerability and emotional numbness, they triggered all the old memories of obsessively checking for lumps, worrying before every check up and interpreting every ache and pain I experienced as an indicator that the cancer had returned.

I knew only too well that I could not underestimate the long-term effect of such mental turmoil. I had to find a way to rectify the situation as I was getting very little sleep. I had no time to waste because I was spending night after night tossing and turning. Even when I managed to drift off to sleep, it was rarely for longer than an hour at a time. It was one of those awful ironies, I couldn't sleep because I was worried and yet I knew I needed sleep or the situation would get worse. I craved sleep because it was the only time I was free of these terrible worries. Yet when I did manage to fall asleep, the following morning it was like waking up to a nightmare. I would wake with my heart racing, totally exhausted and feeling completely desolate.

On the face of it, I managed to go through the motions of looking after the children and keeping the house going, but I knew my feelings of despair were escalating, especially in those small hours of the morning just before the children woke. I would wander around the house as if I was sleepwalking and I have lived to know that the darkest hours really are just before dawn, when every iota of logic disappears.

During these periods of distress, I would get panicky and start fretting, and however much I rationalised with myself that worse things could have happened, and that I was lucky it wasn't worse, I was not consoled. Believe me, it's hard to relax with something like that hanging over you. You try not to spend time worrying, but you just can't help it. You begin to imagine the worst and, before you know it, you have worked yourself into a state.

Even though I was beginning to feel overwhelmed by all this fretting, with my nerves starting to get the better of me, I decided that suppressing these emotions, and not expressing them in an open honest way could be detrimental at this point. Despite the fact that I was wound as tightly as a spring and had no concept of how I was going to shake off this incessant torment, I desperately needed to get to grips with, and defeat, this internal turmoil.

I had so much to live for that I reached the point where I was not prepared to let these unruly, negative thoughts take over my life. The situation was not going to rectify itself, that much I knew, and if my fear was left unchecked, there was no doubt that anxiety and depression could set in.

I did not want to resort to sleeping tablets or other suppressive drugs, even on a short-term basis, as I felt they would only mask the symptoms. I was also concerned that they would create more side effects that might expose me to further trouble down the road. I had had my share of mind-altering drugs the first time I was treated for cancer, when I lived on large amounts of steroids daily. I experienced a ton of adverse reactions to those drugs: half my body seized up, my joints became stiff and immovable as the cortisone seeped into every joint in my body, right through to my fingers and toes – the side effects were endless.

Those drugs messed with my adrenal system terribly. When I was coming off them, I suffered withdrawal symptoms as severe as any heroin addict. The hallucinations I suffered were dreadful: I saw people becoming taller and wider as if I was looking in those weird mirrors you see at theme parks and I shrank away from the walls as I imagined objects falling down on me.

Now, I was dealing with chemotherapeutic drugs that had their own extensive list of side effects. On top of that, I had to cope with the full force of the heavy bombardment of radiation treatments. I recognised that it was crucial to find a course of action that would let me re-establish control of my thoughts and feelings and get me back on track. The words my mother had often spoken came back to me: 'God helps those who help themselves.' They served as a beckoning to me that I had to make a conscious effort to get some sort of plan together – nothing too elaborate, something simple that I could follow and fit into my day-to-day routine. The real problem was working out where to start.

I knew nothing about how someone could influence or control their mind, apart from the occasional motivational lecture or psychological book I had read. The problem was that when I had attended these lectures, I had found that I was inspired and on top of the world, but that feeling soon faded. I also felt that practising meditation needed real commitment and thought it would take a lot of time and effort to master. The only guidelines I had were some relaxation techniques I had learned some years earlier when I practised yoga. As I had nothing to lose, I decided I would start there.

I used the relaxation techniques I knew to help improve my sleep. While I lay in bed, I consciously calmed myself by breathing deeply. When I had begun to relax, I concentrated on tensing and then relaxing the muscles of my body, starting at my feet and working up to my head. This technique is a standard relaxation method taught in any yoga group. As I shifted my attention to each muscle group, I felt a sense of calmness and would drift into a deep sleep.

I must admit that, at first, things were a bit trial and error but, gradually, I began to notice how my sleep improved when I practised regularly. Once I mastered the technique, my sleep returned to normal. I realised I could use this technique on other occasions when I was anxious, like waiting for test results or going back into the hospital for more treatments.

It was a reliable marker for me, that I had the ability to improve my mental state, and I decided I would build on these encouraging results and seek out some other methods such as guided visual imagery to give me back my peace of mind.

Guided Visualisation

Although I have always tried to keep an open mind, I had never been too interested in new-age philosophies, possibly because they symbolised a lifestyle that did not interest me. What I discovered was that these techniques were far from my perception of what was 'new age'; in fact, they were time-honoured practices that took full advantage of mind-body interactions.

I decided to take some instruction from an experienced psycho-therapist. Mary was a devoted teacher with a formidable intellect who was trained to deal with all types of problems – a skill I greatly admired. Her abilities had been highly recommended to me by a trusted friend. She could not have been perceived as self-serving or materialistic as she volunteered her time to help people reshape their lives after facing some crisis or other. I was not sure what to expect, but I had high hopes that this deeply sensitive woman would set me on the right path and make an immense difference to my well-being.

I told Mary that in spite of the fact that I was in the middle of a crisis, I desperately needed to get things into perspective. She reassured me that that was exactly what we would be working towards achieving. Mary provided the necessary support by using guided imagery, a simple non-invasive way of healing that is used to bring about a state of focused concentration. It is used as a standard complementary therapy to help reduce pain, anxiety and the length of stay among the cardiac surgery patients at the Inova Hospital Centre, West Virginia, in the US.

I had read about the benefits of this comprehensive coping strategy some years earlier in Andrew Weil's book *Spontaneous Healing*, a seminal read of my early learning after my first diagnosis. Guided visual imagery is designed to use the power of thought to influence psychological and physiological states. This, in turn, enables relaxation and produces a sense of physical and mental well-being. There is substantial research documenting the effectiveness of guided imagery in changing attitudes towards healing (see the Further Reading section for recommended books on this subject). You may think that you would need a fertile imagination for this type of therapy, but it's not that difficult, as I found when I tried it. To me, it offered good assistance and elevated me from the mental anguish that had been haunting me at the time.

Mary began by outlining what the visual imagery process involved and gave me the details of how it worked. She explained that she would give guided instructions and asked me to visualise them in as much detail as my mind could conceive. She advised me that the more outrageous the image, the stronger the impression it would make on my mind. In my enthusiasm, I fired a volley of questions at her, and she responded by giving me a broad indication of what she hoped I would achieve by the end of the first session. I felt reassured, as she explained that we were not subject to time and there were no rights or wrongs about how I reacted. She made sure we would not be interrupted and I sat back in a comfy chair and we began.

She asked me to create a mental picture of a place where I felt safe, comfortable and relaxed. In my mind's eye, I imagined myself on a family holiday walking down a grassy bank onto a golden, sandy beach. It was similar to a holiday we had been on the previous year, but the setting was a beautiful, tropical beach. Julie my youngest daughter was at that magical age where you want to stop the hands of the clock. I walked along the golden, sandy beach and met up with my husband Ger who was playing with Julie. He had buried her in a hollow that he had dug in the sand. She protested as he slowly sculpted the sandy mound into a mermaid's tail. I reached down and helped her out of the soft, warm sand.

Mary then directed me to focus on sounds, smells and anything that would evoke my senses and make the picture come alive. The water was crystal clear; I was mesmerised by its spectacular colour. I began chatting with Ger as we strolled in a leisurely way along the water's edge. A little girl skipped past us carrying a bucket full of shells, my son and older daughter, Richard and Sarah, came along bearing armfuls of seaweed, and ran after Julie teasing her with the brackish fronds. All of us were in high spirits as Julie screamed in mock terror. I could feel the warmth of the sun, the sand between my toes, the splashing and ripples of the waves coming ashore and, best of all, I could hear the carefree laughter of our children in the distance. It could not have been more perfect as we relaxed under a huge parasol on the beach, watching Richard and Sarah build a great fortresses and a dugout in the sand for Julie while she ran in and out of the white foaming waves. My imagination painted an idyllic picture of that moment that was fuelled with emotion. A sweet contentment washed over me; once again I wanted to freeze the moment and stay just as we were.

I can best describe it as a daydream, but with much more detail than I would normally imagine. I was also able to remember every minute detail afterwards, unlike a dream where you only remember flashes. It was so vivid, I actually felt I had been on holiday, I remember joking with Ger afterwards that it was the cheapest holiday I had ever had. For a first attempt, the depth of the detail I had managed to conjure up surprised me. Best of all was the fact that Mary had restored my confidence in my ability to regain control.

Over the coming months, I returned to Mary and my tropical paradise many times. While I was receiving radiotherapy, I used guided imagery to escape my apprehension and concerns about the effects of the 25 sessions of radiation I was facing. It proved a very useful tool in helping me to stay relaxed and confident that I would soon be on the mend. I promised myself that when the treatment was over, we would all head off to the sun and, to my delight, we recreated my tropical paradise for real. Ger and I exchanged knowing smiles throughout that holiday as we remembered the wonderful daydream I had shared with him on so many occasions during my treatment.

I inadvertently set myself the goal of fulfilling that dream and I guess the anticipation of that lovely holiday helped me to overcome the situation I was dealing with at the time. Remember Dr Waitley's work with the Apollo programme that was mentioned in Chapter 3? 'When you visualize, then you materialize.'

It was a real eye-opener for me to learn how to draw on the powerful potential of my subconscious mind.

In some way, that experience was like lifting a veil. It was not as out of the ordinary as a trance or an unusual state of consciousness would have been. I simply learned how to focus my attention so that I was in control of my thoughts and that was a literal life saver for me.

Over time, I learned to expand the period of focus and build on the positive results I was experiencing. Gradually, as I regained control, my anxieties began to melt away, my spirits lifted and I felt that I was now really starting to get back on track.

It was another major turning point for me as I realised my restored sense of psychological well-being was no coincidence. I had now discovered that it was possible to promote the healing activity of not just the physical body but also the mind. Most of all, I had learned that peace comes from within and that by not ignoring the mental capacity for healing, I had greatly improved my chances of recovery.

So where does that leave those who believe that emotions do not affect the physical body? Most of us need proof before we really believe in something we cannot see. Our social conditioning that 'seeing is believing' is very powerful and yet love is invisible and nearly every human being on the planet believes in it! The love for a child, a lover or a parent cannot be seen, it is an emotion that can only be felt and expressed.

Sex and the Mind-Body Connection

If you still have reservations and still need to be convinced about how strong these mind-body interactions are, take a look at the area of sexual fantasy. Visual images that turn people on and off demonstrate undeniably the powerful connection between mind and body.

Many people engage in sexual fantasy at some stage in their lives. Men and women use their imaginations to tap into visual images that create a highly charged response. The instant physical reactions to the images conjured up during sexual fantasy release neocortical chemicals. Hormones relay electrical signals to part of the brain's hypothalamus, which regulates many processes within the body. This part of the brain is associated with sexual arousal. As arousal intensifies, hormonal responses create an overwhelming euphoria. The strong chemical 'rush' that comes from the release of dopamine and serotonin, two naturally occurring brain chemicals, is widely recognised by neuroscientists.

In their book *Sex Health and Happiness*, Drs Brian and Anna Marie Clement noted that guided imagery could heighten sexual awareness. They cited the findings of Professor Beverly Whipple of the College of Nursing at Rutgers University, New Jersey, in the US. Professor Whipple had conducted research on a group of women who had experienced spinal injuries and paralysis as a result of gunshot wounds, and showed that some of these women could climax through imagery alone.

The authors noted that while this was a new area of research, it offered hope of renewed sexual functioning for those who have been paralysed, and gave the rest of us reassurance that the mind can be a powerful orgasmic trigger.

According to the authors, the mind can literally reprogramme groups of cells in the body to alter their expression and function and directly influences our ability to feel desire. As evidence of this statement consider how powerful imagery has been in your own sex life.

Now consider whether you are prepared to expend that same mental energy on more mundane tasks, such as positive thinking and lifestyle changes.

From Fear to Great Heights

I also had the most wonderful results with visualisation when I used the same technique to conquer my fear of heights. Many of us have some type of phobia – a fear of flying, of elevators, of tunnels, of spiders. Mine was heights. I had struggled with a nerve-wracking fear of heights since I was a young child, and no matter how illogical this may seem, it was a very real fear for me.

Compared to battling cancer, it's not such a major problem but I had missed out on many an adventure over the years because I could not get to grips with it. I had no clue how it started but, as Mary wisely pointed out, we are not born with these fears, we learn them from parents, siblings, teachers or friends. These people have a very strong influence on us when we are young and developing our identities. Mary explained that repetitive fears are normally associated with past experiences, and we react in a similar way because the experience fires the same neuro connections.

Every experience you have is stored in your memory and, along with it, is the emotion of that experience. Fear especially leaves a strong imprint in your memory and, from time to time, certain things trigger the memory of that fear. Not all of our experiences have a dramatic effect on our lives but if they are associated with strong emotions, they can govern our lives. Mary was keen to identify how my fear had started, believing that by understanding and piecing together the past, I could change my negative emotional states. As she began her enquiry with a few pertinent questions, it became clear that this fear came from my childhood.

The memories had faded with time, but when I connected with the problem it was like finding a piece of a puzzle. As I reflected on my upbringing, I had a vague recollection of my mother continually telling me 'You are going to fall' when I ventured to climb the wall outside our house. (Sometimes she was right.) As you may have guessed, Mary explained that this psychological imprinting of a young child (scientifically known as neuro-associative conditioning) can penetrate deep into the sub-consciousness mind and, with time, it becomes deeply ingrained. This type of negative programming can leave us fearful and place restrictions on us that keep us stuck in these limiting beliefs. The more they are reinforced, the more they become ingrained in our belief systems. We may then jump to conclusions if the past associations are negative or faulty.

Mary explained that I had to go back to the original source and reprogramme it to find a better solution. These early childhood experiences can significantly affect our adult lives and this may well have been the link to my irrational fear of heights. It may seem quite simplistic, but somehow discovering how my fear had come about stripped away its hold over me. Over the years, I had allowed this fear to get out of proportion, thinking it was something I would have to learn to live with. Mary thought otherwise. She showed me how to eliminate the mental block and get over this particular mountain. Once again, she pointed out how ignoring what is at your very core can block you from making necessary changes.

Mary asked me to imagine that I was sitting at the top of a Ferris wheel in an amusement park. As I began to imagine myself sitting there, I could feel the gentle breeze rocking the cradle. She then asked me to lift my head and look around. It was a bizarre sensation, just the *thought* of this made my palms sweat and I felt paralysed in my seat. She then asked me to focus on talking to Julie beside me, to imagine we were laughing and having fun. After a short while, I was able to look outside at the surrounding attractions without focusing on the height aspect. This simple coping skill put the mountain I had built up over the years into perspective, and helped me face it.

Chapter Six

Zest for Life

'In health there is freedom. Health is the first of all liberties.'

HENRI FRÉDÉRIC AMIEL

Have you a zest for life or are you stressed with life? If you are stressed, or pushing yourself too hard, taking some time out is not only good for your health, but could also help you rediscover some of life's simple pleasures. In this chapter, I want to point out that if you're going to make it as survivor, you need to connect with what's real in life – with what has substance – and you need to keep away from as many of the persistent stresses of modern living as possible. That means reducing your stress levels and finding ways to re-establish what is really important in your life.

Stress

Stress is a hallmark of the age in which we live; it's like a massive cloud sweeping the globe and appears to be all part of a modern-day's work. The reality is that we find it nigh on impossible to live and work today without experiencing some form of stress.

There has been a sharp increase in stress-related illnesses; absenteeism in the workplace over the past number of years bares testimony to that. As the pace of life becomes more and more frantic, you can see how the upkeep of modern living is significantly affecting us by looking at the people next to you in the train station, the airport and the shops. It is visible on their faces. Stress is all around us: our phone helplines are buzzing with people who are desperate and there is so much written about stress – stress hormones, stressful life events and all manner of ways of dealing with stress – that it's difficult to pick up a newspaper or magazine today without some reference to the stresses of our modern lifestyle. There are many people who never ask for help, those who soldier on and suffer in silence and allow the stress in their lives to grow and grow until they reach breaking point.

We are told that a certain amount of stress is good for us, but it's hard to make clear distinctions between good stress and bad stress. Stress is more than an unpleasant fact of life. When we are stressed we stop looking after ourselves properly – we miss meals, we don't sleep properly, we forget to drink enough water, we have no time to exercise, we may keep ourselves going with sugary snacks, alcohol and cigarettes, and perhaps even drugs. The busy and pressured lifestyles many of us are leading are far more demanding than we realise, and they pose a very real health risk.

When we are subjected to stress, our bodies are pumping adrenalin consistently, which keeps us in a fight or flight mode (the response when danger threatens). The consequences of this response are a poor immune system, poor sleep patterns, poor digestion and impaired memory. There is concrete evidence that shows living in this survival mode can change our biochemistry and suppress our immune systems.

If you want to get away from the stress response and enter into a healing response, you need to look at tackling the amount of stress in your life.

One question I am asked repeatedly is whether stress can cause cancer. Dr Carl Simonton wrote extensively about the strong link between stress and illness (more details about Dr Simonton are given in Chapter 9). Prior to facing a second recurrence of cancer, two things happened in my life that took me way off the stress scale. The first was that my mother had a stroke. When you have an elderly parent, you expect to hear news like this all the time, but it was still a shock when it happened. Fortunately, my mother recovered but she was unable to live alone afterwards. Then, not long after this, my oldest daughter Sarah was diagnosed with a cyst in her brain.

She had been complaining of a headache, which I thought would pass presuming she was coming down with flu or something. But when she complained that both of her cheeks were numb, I realised she had a problem that clearly was not going to go away. A tangible sense of fear started to creep up on me, as I tried to figure out why she had gone numb down one side. Suddenly I was worried, I grabbed her coat, bundled her into the car and rushed to A&E.

As I watched her lying in the hospital bed, ghost-pale and defenceless, I tried to figure out what the problem could be. Could it be something serious? She was only 15 – surely she was much too young to have anything life threatening. It turned out that Sarah had an arachnoid cyst on the left anterior wall of her brain, which, the doctors said, was possibly left over from the embryonic stage. Because of the cyst's location, they decided not to remove it. In all, she was in hospital for nine days. Overwhelmed with relief, we left the hospital. As I sank into bed that night, I thanked God fervently for answering my prayers and keeping her safe and well.

One month later, I discovered a lump in my breast.

Was it a coincidence that I developed cancer a month after these distressing ordeals?

Dr Simonton stated that most of his patients who go through the process of self-examination, see important links between their emotional states and the onset of their disease. 'The process of identifying the links between stress and illness is valuable for everyone, because the link between emotional states and disease applies to susceptibility of all illnesses, not just cancer.'

One exercise that Simonton asked his patients to complete is to list the major life changes or stresses that were going on six to 18 months prior to the onset of their illness. Simonton explained that, 'Most people find when completing this exercise, that the period before the onset of the disease held a number of major stresses.'

In his book *Getting Well Again*, Simonton wrote that:

> *The object of this kind of self-examination is to identify the beliefs and behaviours that you want to change now. Because*

these beliefs have been threatening your health they need to be consciously examined with an eye toward altering them.

Dr Simonton believed that people often place themselves in stressful situations, by putting everybody else's needs first, by failing to say no, or by ignoring their own mental, physical and emotional needs.

Incorporating changes to restore some balance into your busy life will help you cope more effectively with stress and help you appreciate the good things in life. Below is my list of some simple methods to control and relieve stress in our lives today.

Take a Break from Shopping

This may seem like a frivolous stress release, especially when so many of us enjoy the heady endorphin rush we get when we shop, but there are many negative consequences to shopping too much. The stress created by financial woes and the pressures of our consumer society place on us are very real. A friend of mine was one of those who ignored her emotional needs and, instead, became dependent on her 'comfort buys' for emotional support.

Shopping is high on my list as one of today's most common stressors. Any shopaholic will testify to this. Let me be clear, I am not anti-shopping, but I am against the stress that results from society's constant pressure on us to consume. Now I will be the first to admit that I have been known to give into the temptation of a bit of 'retail therapy' – shopping has its virtues. For many women, it relieves the humdrum tedium of domesticity and work. It can be a pick-me-up that has a certain magic about it. But a vital point to consider is whether we are victims of consumerism?

The desire to look good is something that any woman can relate to but when acquiring the latest trend comes at any cost and becomes a compulsion, the joy is short lived and gives way to a habit, or simply satisfying a need. What we, the unsuspecting public, forget to challenge is the all-important question of whether we should buy into the lifestyles that the magazines, television programmes and advertisements bombard us with every day. I understand how easy it is to get caught up in splurging on labels and gadgets. As my shopaholic friend put it, 'When I get what I want, I just want something else. I am a slave for shoes.'

Spending became an addiction for her; she was hooked on buying 'things'. But who could blame her when there are so many of these indulgent goodies up for grabs. Shopping addictions are some-times the result of clever marketing. Advertisers lure us into thinking we need the latest trendy fashions, ruinously expensive age-reversing beauty products, the latest mobiles or gadgets, even silly ring tones and, of course, labels, labels, labels. If you think you are immune to the marketing machine of 21st-century capitalism, think again. You don't get off that lightly, as the engine that drives the wheels of commerce uses subtle psychology to draw us towards wanting trappings of wealth. You have to hand it to them, advertisers are masters at figuring out the psychological value of their products, but this type of media attention has a lot to answer for, as it is fuelling a culture of image-conscious, materialistic people.

Of course companies that create the things we buy are in business to sell and are motivated by profit. Their job is to focus on making money; mine is to focus on health for, without health, you cannot live a normal, fulfilling life.

Shopping has it highs but it also has its downsides. My shopaholic friend is dear to me and much as I like her style, it became apparent that her love affair with shoes and endless shopping sprees were creating a ton of stress in her life. Her spiralling shoe habit took its toll on her relationship. Her 'guilty pleasure' – as she referred to her need to shop – was of little consolation when angry outbursts broke out between her and her husband. Her spending sprees were responsible for much of the tension in their lives and it was beginning to drive a wedge between them. He was completely frustrated with her splurging on designer labels and buying on impulse. Credit card payments were a constant worry for him. I am not sure if she was oblivious to their economic situation or just living in financial denial of their ever-increasing overdraft. Exhausted and elated, she shopped to cover up the uncomfortable feelings of her stressful home life, hoping that a bit of retail therapy would make it all go away.

Despite the fleeting joy that she got when she purchased a fabulous new pair of killer heels, financing her lifestyle produced enormous amounts of pressure. Her excessive dependency on shopping eventually resulted in her completely losing track of the good things in her life – she was so wrapped up in the things she wanted that she barely noticed the things she had. It is an indictment of our modern society that we feel the key to a richer life is all about keeping up with the Joneses. And yet, friendship, love, family, connections with others and self-esteem, are more valuable than some of our most treasured possessions.

I did not want to take sides or get caught up in the turmoil of my friend's domestic difficulties; I am not an expert in sorting out financial woes. Simple logic told me that her obsession with shopping was only fulfilling a purpose, or hiding an emotional need. Lurking beneath her glam exterior was the desire for other people's approval. Social desirability is important to the majority of us and shopping is symbolic of class. Regardless of our background, bigger and better is equated with success, achievement and good performance.

I asked her if all this splurging was making her happy. She looked around suspiciously, then leaned over and whispered, 'Not really, but strange things happen to my reasoning when I see a pair of designer shoes on sale. I know I am a sucker but I just have to have them. Besides I always feel like I am missing out on something if I don't go shopping.'

Apart from the fact that she was up to her eyes in unnecessary debt, the other factors resulting from her 'guilty pleasure' were the mood swings and irritability she displayed when she wasn't shopping. Her lack of motivation for any sort of activity besides shopping was a sure sign of her addiction. I tried to persuade her that material wealth does not always equal happiness. For me, the best way to be happy is by making someone else happy; it is in giving that I feel inner happiness. With it comes satisfaction, purpose and feelings of fulfilment, believe me these are much better motivators; they are the fuel of a richer life.

To tone down her zeal for shopping, my friend had to find some way to get beyond the barriers of self-image. Obsessing over the 'must haves' served several psychological functions for her. Focusing on material things made her feel good and fulfilled her need for approval, it was a substitute for affection and it masked the fact that her marriage was laced with tension.

I wondered if she was a lost cause or if she could find a way of controlling her spendthrift impulses. After some gentle prodding from yours truly, she took the time to see a financial expert who helped her make adjustments to her budget. To help her exercise a bit more restraint, he got her to list her priorities and, together, they devised a sensible financial plan that she felt she could stick to.

I can't say that she is no longer a 'fashion victim' as looking good and having the right image are still very important to her, but my friend has now widened her horizons. She has become less wasteful and a little more concerned with her family and the environment. Appreciating life's simpler pleasures appears to have added more substance to her life. She has taken the first step by breaking her shopping habit and her next challenge is to address the reasons for her compulsion to shop, and to work on the emotional aspects of her life that she has been avoiding.

Try a News Holiday

My second pet hate is the constant tide of bad news we listen to on a daily basis. The media – especially the 24-hour news channels – give so much hype and attention to negative information and we the viewers go through the motions of collectively participating in, listening to and watching it over and over again. Ask yourself: What is your reaction to this endless stream of unpleasant information? Do you get caught up in the dramas and spend time agonising over world events that you are powerless to change? If I were to hazard a guess, I would think your reaction is most likely is that you debate, dwell on and ponder ways that these problems could be solved.

Bad news sells, it is compulsive viewing. The shock of an earthquake that affects thousands can have a profound effect on our mood and behaviour. Our propensity to dwell on this type of news continually penetrates into the mind. *Remember that negative thinking is just as powerful as positive thinking.*

Rather than getting involved in the relentless coverage of negative information, how about doing something to make a difference such as making a donation, volunteering for a relevant charity, or simply vowing that you'll appreciate your own good fortune. Once you've taken action, any action, you no longer feel so powerless; you feel more in control when you make a difference.

In an effort to take the unrelenting bad news out of my day-to-day routine, I have adopted some incredibly easy coping strategies that I have added to my stress-free timeout. A news holiday is a great way to cut loose of the excessive focus on negative events. I have to confess that this drives my husband crazy and he says I am ill-informed about world affairs, but, to be honest, I really don't need to witness acts of violence, terror, war and crime in my living room every evening. I certainly find it difficult to be on the receiving end of this doom and gloom 24/7. If you too feel daunted or bombarded by the constant tide of bad news, you may need some news management:

- You could limit yourself to listening to one episode of the news each day.

- You could switch off the television at news time or switch to your favourite programme.

- Maybe you could create a network of *good* news. My local radio has started a good news slot that cheers me up no end. The internet also has a few sites devoted to good news – who knows, it might catch on.

Take Time Out from Technology

Technological progress has undoubtedly contributed to our stress levels. So intense is the popular interest in new technology that research now shows that we are addicted to surfing the net, social networking, emailing and texting. This is not an overstatement – many psychologists are recognising that internet addictions contribute directly to behavioural problems, sleep disturbances, neglect of studies and work, and muscular and vision problems. Hard-core addicts have problems interacting socially. These net-frazzled fanatics become neurotic and often drop out or withdraw from real life.

The question is this: Is technology bad for your health? Well as technology slowly gains ground in our lives, it brings a new level of anxiety. Shutting out the volume and strain of the overload of information we have to contend with can be difficult.

Not only are the habitual distractions of constant communication stressful, they are also time consuming. The number of work hours wasted by employees surfing the net has come under intense scrutiny by many employers. Monitoring and managing overuse has led many companies to implement measures to restrict, or completely stop, employees access to non-work-related websites.

Even though the web is an excellent tool and resource for researching all manner of information, many of us can find ourselves guilty of excessive use. Entertaining yourself by catching up with friends on Twitter and Facebook may seem like a harmless activity, but this form of online interaction can prevent you from focusing on the important things around you, such as your family, work, outdoor activities or even going to bed. Bloggers' addictions have been known to keep people up all night.

Another aspect of this age of computers and mobile phones is the urge to get connected. Because tech fans are so enthusiastic, they shy away from the thought of being unplugged from their phone or computer. A computer addict needs to be near an internet-enabled device for the majority of their day or they become restless. Many literally suffer withdrawal symptoms because technology controls their life.

Avoiding technology is not an option for many people especially if your job centres on it. However, if you want to make sure that technology does not take over your life you could set up some communication restrictions:

- Discipline yourself to check and answer e-mails only at scheduled times. This will let others recognise the time periods that you are generally available. Parents often allot limits to the time they allow their children to go on the internet and, likewise, you can monitor and discipline yourself so that you don't become hooked. If you struggle with self-discipline, there are software programs that offer visual and audible warnings to alert you when your time is up.

- You may also wish to put boundaries on the time people can contact you by phone. That way, you can reduce your mobile phone dependence. It will also lessen the constant desire to check if you have missed any calls or messages every time your phone beeps. As you gradually begin to adapt, you will lose the urge to be connected.

Give yourself a bit of respite from the constant distractions of technology. I certainly found that not focusing on the internet or emails gave me more time to deal with my busy routine. Once you stop processing masses of data, you reap substantial health benefits. There are psychological benefits from a bit of solitude, and taking time out can alleviate stress and anxiety and help you process your thoughts and ideas more clearly. It can also help you appreciate the good things that life has to offer. With a little down time, you will have much more time for some positive pleasures in your life. So take a break from all that multitasking for even a day or so – I guarantee you will want to keep it up.

Treat Yourself

My favourite stress release that gets me away from my inbox and consistent decision-making is to sit in my garden with a nice cup of tea and take a few minutes out to soak up the atmosphere.

Changing your immediate environment can change your perspective on stressful issues and events. You move into a different mindset when you connect with nature. Modern lifestyles have separated man from nature, yet the research clearly shows that connecting with nature relieves stress and helps restore a sense of calm to our lives. Abraham Maslow believes that humans need aesthetically pleasing imagery to refresh them.

Seeing the beauty in nature has become quite important to me. I have come to value the first snowdrops of spring, the fragrant scents of summer, the explosions of colour that autumn brings and even the crispness of a cold winter's day. Why it has such significance for me now I am not sure. Maybe I have just reached a stage in my life where I could enjoy and experience it.

If you are finding it hard to get a minute's peace, creating a shift in brain activity can clear the mind and provide a nice opportunity to help your brain chill out:

- A good rule of thumb is to allocate a bit of time each day to appreciate and observe your surroundings. It gives you the incentive to get things done and it also creates a nice bit of respite from the demands of a busy day.

- A simple tea break outside can help you relax, unwind and escape from irrelevant bits of information. What could be more relaxing than to stop and sit for a few moments and savour the soothing flavour of a simple brew? Herbal teas have a calming effect and induce relaxation almost immediately. I use chamomile or mint – I have some mint growing in my garden which is wonderfully refreshing. I take full advantage of a little quite time like this; it can offer a wonderful breathing space and bring about a sensation of harmony to my day.

- If you are the get up and go type, exercise can be an important stress buster. It is widely agreed that exercise diffuses pent up aggression and stress. For some, it's a power walk; for others it's a game of golf or tennis. I swear by my early morning walk on the beach, I feel re-energised and rejuvenated afterwards.

Unwind and Meditate

Another release that provides great relief from stress is meditation. It is a wonderful antidote to our noisy, busy lives. I use it to grab a few quite moments when I have spent long hours sitting in front of the computer. People have many questions about meditation and it is a subject they often want to talk about during my workshops and talks. Does mediation really make much of a difference? Can you stop the mental chatter of a busy mind? Is it difficult not to get distracted?

First of all, yes, it works because it releases many of the side effects of stress. When I integrated meditation into my life, it impacted on me in several ways: my sleep improved, my stress levels were reduced and I became more connected with myself and, subsequently, I began to feel more balanced within myself.

The primary reason why meditation contributes to reducing stress levels is that it gives a general sense of calmness and control. Apart from strengthening your body's self-healing powers, it is also a useful tool to have in times of need as it stops the overwhelming feeling of panic that comes when things go wrong in our lives.

Meditation is not a practice that requires you to sit in the lotus position for hours until you reach some kind of advanced Zen state. Even in the absence of any formal techniques, meditation can be carried out quite simply. It is a skill that can be learned easily and carried out where ever you are.

Basically, you can meditate by just being quiet and focusing your attention onto your breath. While the main purpose of meditation is to still the mind, it can also teach you gentle control and use of the breath. Repeating mind-focused breathing can be very beneficial and it is the most basic form of meditation. As your system slows down, you will notice the tension in your body release as you breathe more deeply. When you become focused on the autonomic functions of breathing, you can reduce repetitive thinking. If you are constantly turning things over in your mind, this provides a nice bit of a break. As calmness replaces the constant mental dialogue, it leads to a deeper level of relaxation.

It is universally acknowledged that when you train your mind to abandon the inventory of thoughts you process every day, you begin to unwind. Each day, we generate thought after thought, roughly about 60,000 – and that is a heck of a lot of thinking. The value of shutting down this constant internal noise is that it helps us to engage with ourselves and our lives on a closer level. Quietening the mind stimulates repair mechanisms. Research from Boston University's School of Medicine shows that people who practise yoga have 27 per cent more amino butyric acid in their brains than those who don't, which makes them less susceptible to stress and anxiety, as both these things can be caused by having low levels of this acid.

Neuroscience has found that meditation has the ability to change the structure of the brain. Just 12 minutes a day of relaxation and focused attention can stimulate the frontal lobes of the brain, which is the part that governs our intelligence. Modern technology enables us to see which parts of the brain are activated when we meditate. Meditation puts the rational thinking part of the brain to sleep and reduces the mental chatter. Apart from releasing tension and helping you relax, mediation can help reduce blood pressure and increases blood flow to the brain, which increases oxygen levels. Neuroscience has caught up with the millions of people who believe that meditation benefits the body's natural healing mechanisms.

While it is desirable to practise meditation, most people find it hard to stop their mind from wandering. Creating tranquillity and relinquishing your awareness from the moment-to-moment stresses of life may not always quite flow the way you want it to. Of course, it's easy to get distracted and you are more than likely going to wander off, it is quite normal to observe your thoughts. Seasoned meditators call this the monkey mind because it jumps all over the place, they know that to truly focus your attention, you must park the monkey mind for a few minutes and surrender the need to question, analyse and judge every thought that passes through your mind.

- Disruptive thoughts often challenge your time spent meditating, these responses are habitual. Focusing on them will only make you feel tense, so don't judge yourself for letting your mind wander. God knows it hard enough to get a bit of peace and quiet, don't waste your few quiet moments doing battle with yourself. Instead of turning things over in your mind, turn your attention back to your breathing, when practised regularly, simple meditation techniques will help you find that place of peace where your body can heal. I use a combination of deep breathing and counting backwards from 10 during meditation. Repeating this technique once or twice each day will help you lay the foundation for a lifetime of inner tranquillity and help you rebalance the chemistry of your body to counter the stress and tension in your life.

- I have read a lot of books that discuss the different methods of meditation and while they gave me a foundation of understanding, I realise that some people find it hard to put the theory into practice. From a practical standpoint, I think audio CDs work better for those who want to begin a daily practice of meditation. They give clear explanations and lead the meditation in a way that gives guidance to a novice. The value of this type of instruction is that it helps to build your own practice and enhances your overall experience. If you don't have a CD, play some calming music and focus on its soothing sound, those unwanted thoughts will soon drift away.

There are over 1,500 peer-reviewed studies on the benefits of meditation. If you still have doubts about pursuing meditation, do it for a period of five to seven days. You should find that your body and mind become more energised and that your concentration improves and that your stress levels are reduced. The benefits of mediation are many, but the real way for you to grasp its significance is to try it.

Keep a Journal

Since time immemorial, great philosophers have kept diaries that have charted the events in their lives. What started out for me as a vague notion when I received a gift of a beautifully bound journal has created a much-needed space to unwind at the end of my busy day. I must say I have developed a soothing attachment to writing these pages as I have found it gives me time for reflection.

Although at first I thought it would be a struggle, finding the right words became easy. Sometimes, the pages are dotted with fleeting thoughts that I want to catch before they fade but, for the most part, they are filled with the ordinary events of my family life. Writing these pages is both rewarding and pleasurable and they have formed the seeds of many ideas that have come to fruition for me. I find it insightful and very powerful to record and relive positive events. Day by day, it reminds me not to take for granted the simple, very lovely things in my life and it helps me stay focused on all I have to be grateful for.

Keeping a journal on an ongoing basis can build confidence; we all underestimate our good points, so writing down your strengths increases your self-esteem.

• Setting aside a few moments for you is a good cure for a stressful lifestyle. Many of my readers keep journals and find it a useful tool to express, appreciate and reinforce the good things they have in their lives. The benefit of this exercise is that it helps you to straighten out your thoughts as you relive the events of the day.

- Remember there is no right or wrong way to express yourself, it may be only a few squiggles, but it is a safe and easy way to unlock thoughts and emotions.

Some of my readers find it easier to write in the morning when they are more alert and ideas flow more freely. I find writing in the evening creates a perfect ending to my day. Either way, keeping a journal can create a constructive nurturing dialogue with yourself that provides constant comfort. It also helps you to deal with minor frustrations and can offer a fresh way of relating to others and yourself. In the wider sense, it can help you step back and assess what is important in your life.

If keeping a journal does not appeal to you, then perhaps some other creative outlet might. It is a great release to become absorbed in something creative. It doesn't have to be limited to painting and sculpture. It can be as sedate as knitting or as active as building a tree house. There is great satisfaction in creating something with your own hands. These activities rebalance our brains, whose logical left side is typically over-stimulated. Try it – you may find it stimulates your creative side. If you prefer to be doing something to unwind, some sort of mental activity might work better for you. It could be a crossword, Sudoku, brain training, bridge or attending a course. It can be absolutely anything so long as you find it mentally relaxing.

Connect with Friends

This is my all-time favourite way to relive stress. Spending time with friends is a great way to deal with the dilemmas and emotional upheavals of life. Having a laugh is an instant, natural mood elevator that releases endorphins (health-enhancing hormones) and creates more serotonin (a neurotransmitter that helps combat stress). Stress-reducing humour has both physiological and psychological benefits. They say that laughter is the best medicine, but the beauty of a good laugh is its contagious, such is the magic of laughter that the chances are you won't be able to stop yourself joining in. As the old Irish proverb says, 'A good laugh is the best cure in the doctor's book.'

Even the anticipation of a good night out can lift your spirits and create a general feeling of well-being. Sharing time with friends not only elevates your mood but it also takes the focus away from yourself and can give you a light-hearted perspective on problems.

Friends often know you better than you know yourself and can help you view things in more positive ways. A good friend can give you confidence, help you through a crisis, deflect negative criticism or just be there for you when you need them. This provides a support system that helps you cope with stress or difficult life experiences.

Of course things can go awry with relationships. Stress, struggling with jobs and family life can all stand in the way of keeping in touch with friends. Stress is notorious for driving people inward and isolating them. Friendships can end or drift apart if we don't cultivate them.

Losing a friend can be really tough because we share a history, interests, pursuits, concerns and successes with them. These common bonds are both enjoyable and important because they fill our lives with meaning and purpose. Yet many of my readers have told me how they have held grudges against friends for years. It may not be his or her fault, but harbouring negativity is not good for anyone's health. One thing I can tell you is survivors don't waste emotional energy holding grudges. It is a great injustice to your health if you cannot mend a broken friendship.

If certain things are frustrating or bothering you about your friends ask yourself what you are going to do about it. If the answer is nothing, then it can't be that important.

Remember when these difficult emotions come to the fore, it's not the end of the world. Don't waste time looking back on the small stuff, life is definitely too short for that. If you want to eliminate as much stress from your life as possible, get out of emotional ruts. Remind yourself of the bigger picture and move on from your incompatibility, and reconnect with your desire for companionship. Real friendship is about giving and expecting nothing in return. Human contact of touch, love and friendship is a priceless gift to give and receive. The benefits are immeasurable, when you share yourself from the heart, you will receive back more than you give.

We can all do with a little help from our friends, so go on get reacquainted with the people you value most in your life.

Focus on the Good in your Life

There is real satisfaction in restoring balance and getting more connected to the good things in life. If you want to turn your life towards physical, mental and spiritual regeneration start by appreciating the things you have.

It is so common to dwell on the things that go wrong in life. If you continually reaffirm negative things about yourself, you become disheartened and discontented. There are countless ways to put the zest back into your life. Pay attention to the things that are essential to your happiness. This should be a priority if you want to shift your focus away from the negative.

- Focus on your achievements because when you focus on what is good and working in your life, it feels good. Focused thinking helps you hone in on your successes, and helps you bring your successes to the surface.

- Clarify your successes. Everyone's definition of success is different – for some it is big, for others it is small. Learn to acknowledge your achievements by writing them down, highlight them, talk about them with your friends and your family, especially your mum, as mothers are only too happy to listen to the successes of their children.

- Take stock of the good things in your life and be thankful for them. Many beautiful things are free to all of us and are very often overlooked or taken for granted.

- If you want to be more positive, avoid negative words like 'I am dying to …' Rephrase the sentence into positive terms such as 'I am looking forward to …' Your words are a reflection of your thoughts, when you create a vocabulary for success by using positive terms, your mind hears positive statements. It makes you more positive and also sets an example for those who surround you as they may also choose a positive vocabulary over a negative one.

Of course, these are just a few practical strategies for dealing with stress, there are many other ways to reduce stress and anxiety, but these simple tactics have been a positive influence in my life and have left me better equipped to handle stress. They are rooted in my conviction that some of the best things in life really are free.

Chapter Seven

Looks can be Deceiving

⌒

'Life's challenges are not supposed to paralyze you, they're supposed to help you discover who you are.'

BERNICE JOHNSON REAGON

Looks can be deceiving and can often mask the dark events that shape our lives. Anyone who has come face to face with any emotional upheaval will tell you, constantly portraying a false exterior, a brave face, can affect your emotional well-being. Some of those I have helped had been tormented because they could not address their fragile emotions. In order to find the root cause of their troubles, I found that I had to dig a bit deeper. I found that life was a constant inner struggle for those who had suffered the ravages of trauma, rejection, betrayal, abuse or abandonment. Whether they had been the victim or the perpetrator, the pain and raw emotion of the trials they had faced turned into barriers to their recovery.

Yet if the root cause of a problem is not treated, the impact and affects of negative feelings and pessimistic thoughts lead to stored anger, blaming, judging, jealousy, vulnerability, control issues and low-self esteem. These negative feelings are carried in our cellular memory and feed anxiety and despair.

Many of the people who came to me for help had sourced outside relief to their problems from medication, because they lacked the coping skills needed for healing. It took a huge amount of courage for them to face the truth, but as the truth is the starting point in any development, many mustered up that courage in order to liberate themselves. When dark thoughts or feelings are a part of your life, you cannot actually experience real health, because these feelings hold you in their grip – like the walls of a prison – and are symptomatic of emotional vulnerability.

'Painful things happen to nearly all of us in life,' says Dr Arthur Janov author of *The Primal Scream*. He has noted how repression sets in to block feelings:

> *They get imprinted in all our systems which carry the memories forward, making our lives miserable. This can create a host of neurotic behaviours and physical symptoms. Our ability to separate ourselves from our feelings is the uniquely human survival adaptation to an overwhelming world. It is almost impossible to eradicate deep depression without plunging into the depths of the unconscious where the basis of it all lies.*

In his book, he concluded by writing that patients can dramatically reduce debilitating medical problems, such as depression, anxiety, insomnia, alcoholism, drug addiction and heart disease by unblocking repressed emotions.

Past experiences often force us to erect emotional barriers. We swallow our tears and cover up our hurt, sadness, anger, failures, guilt and resentments. These emotions lurk at the edges of our consciousness, sometimes nagging at us, as if they are trying to tell us something. Without admitting it, we direct these feelings inwards and banish them to the dark places of our minds, hoping they will not surface again. The problem is that destructive emotions that have been repressed often manifest in illness. When repressed emotions are locked away and have no outlet, they can be the cause of serious physical symptoms. Evidence certainly suggests that unresolved negative emotions can lead to a suppression of the immune system, which may in turn enable disease to invade our bodies.

Negative emotional states have a ripple effect in the body, playing a significant role in increasing susceptibility to disease. They can directly compromise the body's natural defences. Happy thoughts increase the immune-building interferon, interluken and imipramin, whereas unhappy thoughts produce the immune-destroying cortisol and adrenalin.

Since negative emotional states have such a profound effect on the body's ability to heal, it is imperative that these hidden emotions are looked at properly. Now that seems logical – doesn't it? Seeing the truth behind what appears on the surface is a must if you are to identify the cause of any trouble you are experiencing. But we sometimes cannot see the wood for the trees when we are directly involved in problems of this nature. We treat the symptoms but don't identify the cause. This is especially obvious when it comes to identifying why an illness has developed.

Laura's Superficial Façade

The advantage of learning to abandon negative emotions is that it is incredibly liberating. Laura described it like this: 'I know I can't change the past, but letting go of it was like being let out of prison.'

For years, she had been stricken by her own private calamity. Yet her outward appearance belied her troubled emotions. In fact, it was hard to detect in her appearance and demeanour any of the guilt and shame she had concealed for many years.

Consequently, she found herself in a dichotomy of looking one way while feeling quite another. When I first came across Laura at one of my seminars, I was not quite sure what ailed her but I was struck by how deep and intense this beautiful, fair-haired woman was. Some people would say there is a sort of narcissism about people like Laura, she was a flawless beauty and appeared to have everything – but looks can be very deceiving.

Despite the superficial veneer that she tried hard to portray, I sensed that some deep, emotional issue troubled this young woman. Whilst only in her mid-thirties, she had developed heart disease. Knowing only too well that physical symptoms are so often connected to emotional problems, I asked Laura to think back to when the problem had started: was she under emotional stress? Frequently, this gets right to the heart of the trouble and fleshes out the underlying cause of an illness. Her answer contained the usual facts about the cholesterol lowering drugs she had been prescribed, how her cardiologist had said she was in danger of having a heart attack because her scans showed her main artery was 70 per cent blocked and two others had a 60 per cent blockage. She went on to explain how she was advised to have immediate surgery but that she could not bear the thought of the operation. However, she told me nothing about the emotional aspect of her life.

After I had given her some details about the correct foods to stop the build-up of fatty material that causes hardening or furring of the arteries (atherosclerosis), she asked me if coronary heart disease could be arrested or reversed without surgery. As the vast majority of disease results from blocked blood vessels, I explained that heart disease is the hallmark disease of an animal-based diet. Nowadays, many people have woken up to the fact that a plant-based diet can help the body mop-up these fatty deposits in the arteries.

I asked if she was familiar with the work of Dean Ornish, the famous cardiologist who had inspired former US president Bill Clinton to change his diet. Ornish pioneered the reversal of heart disease through diet, exercise and stress management. I explained about the people who participated in his lifestyle intervention programme and their incredible results. Apart from these practical steps, Ornish also emphasises the value of love in health. In his book *Love and Survival*, he proposes that our very survival is dependent on the healing power of love, intimacy and relation-ships. When I mentioned this to Laura, she became anxious to finish our conversation and then walked away quickly. She had an expression that puzzled me. Why did she react so abruptly? Why was she so agitated? What was the cause of her negative reaction? Was it a broken romance, perhaps a trust broken in childhood?

Two weeks later, I received a call from Laura asking if I could help her get to grips with changing her diet. I agreed and, over the coming months, we worked together to improve her lifestyle. Throughout that time, I learned that she had been taking anti-depressants for years. I found this bit of background knowledge worrying, because I knew that in 2005, the American Food and Drugs Administration had adopted a black-box warning label on all anti-depressant medications to alert the public to the potential increased risk of suicide attempts for those taking these drugs. This warning stresses that patients taking anti-depressants should be closely monitored and assessed regularly during treatment. The UK's National Institute for Health and Clinical Excellence (NICE) recommends that people try counselling before they take prescription drugs, which are designed to give people an emotional lift, from their doctor.

Dr Andy Bernay-Roman, author of *Deep Feeling, Deep Healing*, is convinced, after years of working with critically ill patients in intensive-care units, hospices and healing centres, that repressed emotional pain lies at the root of many diseases. 'Thoughts have biological consequences that can construct or destruct health,' he says. A psychologist interested in the whole picture of health, and especially the role that stored, hidden, feelings play in setting the stage for illness, Bernay-Roman believes that if you have symptoms of body or mind, you must find the answers in your unconscious mind. He is convinced that removing the blocks to feeling is the most direct route to re-establishing the biological basis of healing in the body. And that the 'invisible factors' of thoughts and feelings are key to influencing the physical condition.

Because the body reflects the health of the mind, when we battle only the outer effects of a disease, the inner distress experienced during times of crisis can be suppressed.

As past behaviour provides useful clues to understanding our present emotional and mental states, I was hoping that Laura's need for physical health would provide her with a breakthrough from her dark past into a brighter future. Although she gained confidence and trust in our friendship over those months, she was not ready to share her traumatic secret. While teaching, I have seen what holding in emotional pain does to people, and how it shapes their lives in negative ways. Equally, I have seen how fulfilling physical needs can help people override the ghosts of their past and help them to move on to successful lifestyles, relationships and achievements. Sometimes, the answers are on our doorstep but we can't see what is staring us in the face.

I addressed her depression with concern and put the same question to her on many occasions. A bigger question was: What is the cause of your depression? I raised another pertinent question when I asked her what she liked about herself, hoping that her answer would tell me a bit about the way she saw herself and what was at the heart of her problem. This core question would help me understand the way she viewed her life, its purpose was to unmask the picture she wanted to portray. I wanted to get nearer to her and find the real person behind the mask.

She never answered me.

For whatever reason, Laura was overtly suspicious of trusting others. While this may have been the symptom of a painful relationship, it was clear to me that she had a visceral fear of revealing her emotions. Fear of facing unexpressed feelings is a hindrance to emotional health because it stops you seeking help. For Laura, it pushed her beyond her emotional limits.

It took some time to discover how palpable her turbulent childhood was in her present life. When childhood experiences are negative, they can severely damage a child's social development. The first clue I had of the lifelong psychological scars with which Laura had battled was her relationships with members of her family. She had no contact with them, although she spoke affectionately about her younger brother, Andrew.

Trapped in the Past

While she had tried hard not to allow her painful memories to resurface, it became apparent to me that profound emotional isolation had resulted from some early experience in Laura's life. My first insight into her tortured past came on a breezy, autumn day when we went walking by the beach. It was then that I learned of the destructive nature of this woman's childhood that had haunted her well into her adulthood life.

At the tender age of eight, Laura was sexually abused by her mother's brother. This traumatic event turned her world upside down.

She took a deep breath as she said, 'I remember the first time so vividly; it was a Saturday evening and he had come to baby sit me and Andrew. He called me into the bedroom and took off my clothes. I thought he was getting me ready for bed, I didn't really understand what was happening, but it made me feel bad when he pressed his body into me.'

For years Laura had trusted and looked up to her favourite uncle who called regularly with treats, played with her and bought presents at Christmas time. She unleashed a stream of emotions as she recollected how he betrayed her mother's and father's trust.

'I knew deep down inside me it was wrong. Why did I let him do that to me?' she said with anger welling up inside her.

Her problem was not of her making, yet she was punishing herself for crimes she hadn't committed. As she suffered quietly, she desperately wanted to tell her mother about what was happening but he had brainwashed her into believing something bad would happen to her if she told anyone.

It was a frightening, heavy burden for someone so young to bear. Laura learned not to speak a word, but her silence could not dampen the fear, anger and frustration she felt. With no outlet for her pent-up feelings, the young Laura retreated into herself. During this protracted period, she found, deep within herself, an inner source that bridged the gap between fear and endurance.

'How did you feel?' I asked cautiously.

'I felt so alone. There was no one to ask; I had no one to confide in. I felt disconnected, fearful and, most of all, I felt damaged.'

It was hard to imagine the abusive nightmare she had suffered at the hands of a family member. How could he inflict such suffering on a child? I am sure she noticed the flicker of alarm that crossed my face as the extent of the physical torment she went through emerged. It was disturbing to hear how her childhood had been torn apart by this malevolence. Why had this manipulative man free reign over this young child? And why had there been such a lack of supervision from her parents who should have watched out for her welfare?

Surely they must have noticed how he had exploited their child or at least the results of the abuse he had dished out. Looking back, I wondered how she survived in the absence of such support. Unfortunately, this had not been an isolated incident and, throughout the coming years, the abuse had escalated and she had been repeatedly mistreated, often in the room next to her parents. Laura became concerned for Andrew who this man was now beginning to show an interest in.

With good reason, she became suspicious of the cosy relationship this man was developing with Andrew. She remembered Andrew sitting quietly on his lap while he stroked himself. Laura was the only one who knew why Andrew cowered away when their uncle came into the room.

'Needless to say he didn't want to risk exposure so he made sure to cover his tracks,' she said as the fury rose inside her.

His compulsion to control was all too familiar to Laura. Even though, at that stage, she was only 10 years old, it was obvious to her that he was intent on strengthening his foothold in their lives and he was going to great lengths to gain her sibling's confidence. Ever vigilant, she watched on while he carried out the masquerade of being the caring uncle. Determined that he would not force or trick her little brother into any kind of sexual act, Laura did her best to take the focus away from Andrew. Despite the fact that she was scared stiff, Laura surrendered herself to him. Her parents interpreted this as sibling jealousy, but they did not know the silent secret that passed between Laura and her uncle.

'I had to, I couldn't let him do that to Andrew. I had to watch out for him especially when my mother was out working. That was when we really had to fend for ourselves,' she said as she relived the memories.

The fear, meaningless pain and wasted time that she had suffered at the hands of this man was unbearable for Laura, but she was powerless to scare him away. For a long time, she pretended it didn't happen and tried to erase it from her mind. She convinced herself so much that, in the end, she began to wonder if it had really happened at all.

The force of negative emotions can distort memories and, consequently, we find it hard to distinguish truth from lies as we toss them over in circles in our minds. These tricks of the mind can often solidify our belief that things are normal. Sadly, this type of mistaken belief can stop you from identifying these mixed-up feelings and articulating the problems. Laura did not know how to sort out these hidden emotions.

Eventually, she found the courage to speak up, it was her greatest challenge. She recalled the final occasion that he abused her, although unsure of the words she bravely told her mother. It took all her energy to go to her mother that day, she was only 11 years old. She had never before spoken of such things and she didn't know how to explain it.

Her mother was horrified, the truth was inconceivable.

Laura had thought she had done something wrong, that she had disappointed her mother. She had genuinely believed that her mother would turn him over to the authorities, but she had done nothing. She had discreetly brushed it aside and hadn't even told her husband because she knew he had a terrible temper. When her mother had approached her perverted brother, he had taken the moral high ground and, typically, defended his position. He had fabricated a whole story that had painted Laura as jealous and disruptive and her mother had believed him.

The startling conclusion of her attempt to solve the problem had been she was met with a wall of indignation and disbelief. As her life rapidly crumbled around her, Laura had felt betrayed. She gave a brief glance at me as she explained how her childhood had been stolen.

This revelation had broken the bond between Laura and her mother. Ostracised by her mother, Laura had been abruptly moved to a school in the country which was run by nuns. This tough love had been of little consolation to the young and inexperienced Laura. The wrench of leaving her beloved bother had widened the gulf in Laura's struggle and conflict.

Although denied this important relationship in her life, its loss had been overshadowed by the relief of being free of that dark and miserable time. While the sterile surrounding of a boarding school had not been the answer to her problems, her desire for freedom from the fear and anger that had filled her body had far outweighed her need for her brother's affections.

'That was really when I learned to put on a brave face. At times, I found it really hard to control my anger. Can you imagine what it feels like to be angry all the time?' she asked. 'For the most part the convent school was grand, although some of the girls were bitchy. I tried to box the whole thing off, maybe I just was not mature enough to handle it at the time.'

Desperate to heal the shame that had infected her, Laura explained how she had often rationalised the consequences of revealing herself emotionally but felt suspicious and mistrustful of people's reactions. I asked why she had never sought help to deal with these troubling memories.

'I badly wanted to talk about it but where would that get me? Who would I talk to? The girls at school? None of them had ever gone through anything like that, and problems like this were not the kind of thing you talked about then. Besides, it's very hard to bare your soul to a stranger. I couldn't deal with the stigma and shame of opening up that can of worms,' she said.

Laura didn't mention the abuse to her doctor, although she told me that she had often rehearsed what she would say to him. Laura was sure he would think she was some kind of pathetic sympathy-seeker, muckraking up the past. He gave her the pills and that was that.

One of the hardest things to do is to admit that you need help to let go of negative feelings. Laura was simply not addressing the issues she needed to – ironically, suppressing negative emotions helps prolong the hold they have on us. However, there are times when we have to go back in order to change the future.

There are many advantages to laying past traumas to rest, yet we often hang on to our woes, even when we know the negative impact they are having on our well-being. Weary of opening up old hurts, Laura ignored her troubled state of mind. It was much easier to turn her back on these hurts in the hope that the passage of time would dampen their intensity. The result of these untreated wounds was the superficial façade that she put in place. Another consequence of her inability to seek help was that she spent her life pondering the fact that she would be labelled as an abused child.

After she had left school, Laura had a new sense of freedom but the legacy of her childhood gnawed away at her. For a time, her personality reflected the deep-seated anger of her grim upbringing. She didn't make real friends and found it really difficult to form an intimate relationship.

'He screwed me up sexually. If I am honest, it was me who alienated those who tried to get close to me. When I left school, I got in with a bad crowd – believe me I was no angel. I became promiscuous, smoked dope and drank a lot of alcohol, I lived a pretty unhealthy life.'

In a way this covered over the cracks, and, eventually, Laura ended up on 30 milligrams of Prozac, suffering with depression. As the years rolled by, she found solace in the medication and came to depend on it throughout the coming years.

Finding Closure

As her physical health was suffering, I attempted to intervene, hoping that Laura might resolve the conflict inside her. Finding closure for such events is not an easy task, as they leave deep, long-lasting scars. I explained that even though she may find these feelings difficult to articulate, going back to living with the same old problems would not work either. That would only convert the memories into more frustration, disappointment and stress. I tried to convince her that the abuse was only one aspect of her life and there was so much more she could accomplish if she was not paralysed by this trauma. She was trapped in the past and was so fixated on it that she had forgotten about her future. While she found our conversation a great relief, I felt Laura needed more than a friend with a good listening ear to talk with.

There are times when virtual strangers can be of more help than close friends. Competent therapists are trained to spot underlying problems and to offer support and help as they highlight solutions for dealing with these sensitive emotional issues. A trained professional can help you identify the areas that need attention. Laura needed to talk openly and honestly with someone who would understand what she had gone through.

Today, there is an increased acceptance of people taking guidance from a counselling psychologist or life-coach. A counselling psychologist focuses more on psychological, emotional issues, where as clinical psychologists are more medically orientated, focusing on the treatment of disease, for example people with serious mental illness. I want to make this clear because some people still hold on to the belief that you have to be mentally ill in order to seek professional help. This type of misconception can stop people acknowledging their problems and asking for help. Working with a therapist is not something you have to whisper about. Nor is it a sign of weakness.

Opening the lines of communication would be key for Laura to eliminate her fears and self-doubt. She agreed that it was foolish to stay attached to the old hurts and that she badly needed to let go of them. She found it hard to make this move but I assured her there was no need to be embarrassed or fearful. I encouraged her to believe that the time had come to get on with living and think about her future.

In my mind, it is an obvious step to recovery, yet, for the majority of people, the hard part seems to be making the decision to seek help in the first place. I have seen so many good things come when people release the feelings that lie beneath the surface. The benefits of an increased sense of self-esteem, self-worth and self-reliance can boost your confidence no end. It cannot be overemphasised that it is never too late to seek help. There are many programmes designed to break through these boundaries and find what is preventing you from moving on in your life. Remember, they are there to help and support, not to judge and criticise. Seeking help made a crucial difference to Laura's life.

Even though it was perfectly understandable that she would find it hard to move into dialogue and vocalise her feelings, I advised Laura not to let that put her off. The road to recovery is the culmination of many steps along the way; we found a doctor who weaned her off the anti-depressant medication and a reliable therapist named Audrey who Laura seemed to develop a rapport with. We had checked Audrey's qualifications to make sure she had adhered to the accepted ethical standards of practice and, when we were confident that she had all the verifiable data we were looking for, I explained to Audrey that it was imperative that Laura didn't feel pressured. Audrey understood perfectly.

In a professional, discreet manner Audrey set a secure-base from where Laura could disclose the secret she had harboured for so many years. As Audrey tried to reach deep into the depths of Laura's soul and get below the surface, Laura found her probing questions hard to deal with. Nonetheless, as she began to drop her defences, she spilled out her agonising feelings about the violation, separation and anxiety that had been fuelled by her abuse.

Establishing Coping Skills

Audrey facilitated Laura, at her own pace, in establishing coping skills. Laura explained that she often had flashbacks of her abuse. Audrey reassured her that these memories although unsettling were over, that they had happened a long time ago, and none of it was her fault. She advised Laura to visualise a barrier around these negative flashbacks. Imagining a wall between her and what she wanted to keep out made her feel more protected.

Laura took a class in creative visualisation and found that practising the relaxation exercises she learned formed a wonderful connection that nurtured her wounded childhood. Visualising is especially helpful in these situations as the brain thinks in pictures. Imagery can open up paths to the unconscious right brain because emotional responses depend on neuro pathways which link the right hemisphere of the brain to the left hemisphere.

Audrey found various ways to hone in on Laura's needs, and she helped her address her urge to use alcohol as a crutch. Although

Laura had long since given up smoking dope, she spent most nights comforting herself with a bottle of wine, despite the fact that she was taking prescription drugs.

In addition, Audrey helped her create physical boundaries to give Laura a sense of strength. Laura began to wear clothes that made her feel more empowered and give her confidence. She looked fabulous.

As Laura moved through the pain, Audrey began to focus on her strengths and asked Laura to make a list of her strengths and dreams for her future. She discovered that Laura had a deep desire to work with disadvantaged children. Working with under-privileged children was something she had wanted for quite some time but she never had the courage to chase her dream because she felt unsafe. Audrey fostered this interest in Laura because she felt it could be a mechanism for change. Because this resonated deeply with Laura, Audrey asked her to set a target that she would fulfil this dream. She explained that picturing her goal would help her stay focused on materialising her vision, she also pointed out that although the unfamiliar territory of this adventure may seem daunting, knowing what she desired was not enough, she had to take steps down a different path if she wanted to fulfil and experience that dream. This struck a chord with Laura and she seized the opportunity to fulfil her long-time desire.

A Fresh Start

This fresh perspective helped Laura to bring the truth out of the shadows and she found a deep level of personal growth as she reached beyond her normal perception of her damaged life. As she found her footing along her path, she also found an escape route from the familiar disruption of her former lifestyle. The therapeutic benefit of counselling definitely helped her break free of her childhood and all its emotional baggage. As the agony of all those years began to dissipate, the quality of Laura's life improved immeasurably.

It took great courage for Laura to face the underlying issues that she had lived in constant denial for so many years. Letting go of her unresolved emotions was a vital step for Laura; it helped her move on and also stripped away the superficial veneer that she felt she had to wear for the sake of others.

As soon as she began to face her fears, the change was quite rapid. Her new-found freedom correlated with her ability to face her fear and self-doubt and finally get this problem off her chest. Audrey became the principle architect in guiding her back to a state of emotional well-being, while I worked in the background on her diet and physical needs. As soon as her diet brought about positive changes in her blood work, Laura decided against surgery.

In a way, the need for physical change became a form of therapy for Laura. Painful as it was, embracing the overriding need for physical health became cathartic for her. The impending by-pass surgery forced her to focus on not just her present physical needs but also her emotional needs. It somehow put the onus on her to pull herself out of the past and it helped her get rooted in the present. Laura felt blessed to have been given a fresh start and this translated into her finding closure to the difficulties she experienced during her early life.

When she finished her time with Audrey, Laura joined an organisation that works in the world's poorest areas across Asia and Latin America. Helping provide food, shelter, sanitation and love for abused children became a key focus in Laura's life. She found deep fulfilment working and connecting with these children and received much more than she had bargained for as she journeyed through their troubled lives. Devoting her time to their needs provided a better future for her. It was a blessing in disguise. She turned the forces of her abusive past to her advantage and became stronger and more fulfilled because of it. Six years on, she has found it has brought a heightened awareness of her emotional and spiritual being. We humans may be tainted by bad habits, negative thinking and emotional insecurities, but we have also wonderful qualities of love, friendship, support and connection with others.

When she last put pen to paper, Laura wrote:

For the first time in my life I can be myself and it feels good. Søren Kierkegaard said that, 'Life can only be understood by looking backward; but it must be lived looking forward.' If I look back on the bitterness and shame I tried to cover up, I think that is what brought me to the brink of a heart attack. It may sound absurd but maybe that experience was mapped out for me so that I would be able to understand what these children go through. I can't say I value the experience but it has opened a door within me that may have otherwise remained locked. It has helped me become more in tune with myself and the needs of others.

Pursuing her dream was a wonderful way for Laura to assuage the pain of her childhood. The releasing process was a useful tool for change and was a key element in her personal growth. Letting go of the ravages of her past was essential to her regaining control of her emotions, her health and her life.

It is the willingness to let go that is important, the willingness to heal the past. Let me reassure you that you do not have to live your life within negative boundaries. Even if you never consult a therapist, don't let the constraints of old beliefs keep fears, insecurities and limitations in place. Real personal growth comes from letting go, from forgiveness, from loving yourself with all your limitations and past mistakes, loving life and loving others despite their mistakes. Letting go of what lies beneath heals us and gives us an opportunity for a new beginning.

In Laura's case, when she was confronted by what she had perceived to be a life-threatening operation, this somehow helped her to banish the wounds of the past and move on.

Chapter Eight

What Lies Beneath

∽

'A happy life cannot be without a measure of darkness, the word 'happy' would lose its meaning if it were not balanced by sadness.'

CARL JUNG

To develop a survivor's attitude, many of the people from whom I received feedback – the victims of parental disapproval, unresolved grief, serious illness or other traumas – used various therapies that they found were important components of their healing. For some, these therapies provided a breakthrough experience that changed their vision about life; in other cases, it provided a physical relief that proved particularly useful to bring down the walls they had erected around their emotions.

I decided to try one of these therapies for myself in order to give a better picture of how it works.

I had a lengthy interview with a psychotherapist Anthony Chatham. Anthony holds graduate degrees in psychology, philosophy and theology. I explained to him my personal and professional interests in finding avenues for healing debilitating emotions and we discussed how physical ailments are often overshadowed by emotionally charged issues. Anthony explained that when we avoid looking at our emotions, we deny ourselves the power to change our circumstances and put things right. By eliminating the cause, the effects of emotional problems can be dramatically reduced.

Anthony explained that regression therapy is often helpful in these cases. This therapy's scientific grounding is well established and is widely recognised by medical professionals for patients suffering from post-traumatic stress. As a therapy, it is used to bring up traumatic images through eye movement. Reprogramming and desensitisation is used to free the mind of disturbing events and emotions. It is based on the principle that we record and retain all our life experiences in our minds.

Regression Therapy

Regression therapy was developed by psychologist Dr Francine Shapiro who observed that eye movements reduced the intensity of disturbing thoughts (see www.emdr.com). EMDR (eye movement desensitisation and reprocessing) involves recalling a stressful past event and linking with what was felt, seen and believed at the time of the trauma. The therapist induces a pattern of rapid directional eye movements to reprogramme memories. It is believed that rapid eye movements facilitate the neural circuitry of the brain's two hemispheres to work out a co-operative solution to problems. Research on how the eyes track moving objects, carried out at the University of Illinois in Chicago, shows subtle abnormalities in eye movements in schizophrenic patients. Developments in tech-nology can now measure these abnormalities and compare them with normal patterns (see www.ascribe.org).

A new study by researcher Stefan Glasauer, from the Bernstein Centre for Computational Neuroscience and Ludwig-Maximilians University in Munich, about how the brain analyses the speed and movement of an object, shows how the eye adapts to changes in the speed of fast-moving objects more than slow-moving objects, a phenomenon believed to help us gain control.

Although the EMDR treatment has been used widely in recent times, claims of its efficacy have been criticised, yet many practitioners involved in psychiatric nursing find it a viable treatment for their patients that is preferable to psychiatric drugs. Many clinicians have found this element of psychotherapy to be a unique addition in relieving the anxiety associated with trauma. EMDR treatment has been helpful in the treatment of post-traumatic stress, physical or mental abuse, molestation, addictions, insomnia, nightmares, flashbacks and grief issues.

EMDR is more of a non-verbal therapy, which can be beneficial for those who find it difficult to talk about their problems. The techniques used in regression therapy include visual and audio stimulation to guide the conscious mind, enabling the person to reach back into stored memories to any point in life that they want to recall. This is done by engaging the person in a deep meditative state, where they are able to access subconscious or conscious feelings. The therapist provides the format and technique, the individual provides the memories.

Anthony explained that anyone can benefit from these techniques, adults or children, as it is a safe way to connect with unresolved painful emotions. Children are particularly open to this therapy as, unlike adults, they are not as cynical and rigid in their beliefs. Picturing your memories is the main focus for this deep exploration, but auditory direction from the therapist can also help to retrace memories. Throughout the therapy many people recall memories of a loved one, let go of pain, unresolved emotions or discover an aspect of their personality that they had not been aware of.

It is necessary to build trust with a therapist and Anthony's quiet, soothing mannerisms made me feel at ease. His Indian ancestry has inspired him to *focus on wellness, not on illness.* I have highlighted this because it struck me that focusing on wellness could hone in on our strengths and not on our problems. It's a common trait of human nature for the mind to gravitate towards the negative rather than the positive but by focusing on and connecting with our strengths rather than our weaknesses, we can achieve enormous success.

Given the proliferation of new therapies in the field of mental health, I wondered if this therapy could open a window of understanding to the physical and emotional blockages I had experienced in my own life. Always curious and open to different strategies, I decided I would try to evaluate its therapeutic value for myself. For many years after my surgery, I had a painful breast. My doctors told me it was scar tissue or the effects of the radiation treatments I had been exposed to – perhaps regression therapy could be a new way to heal this old wound.

In order to enable me to select the internal response and bring forth memories, Anthony used different procedures of intervention for restructuring emotional blockages, the first of which was following the moving lights on an EMDR light machine until my eyes spontaneously and rapidly shifted back and forth. Therapists often use their fingers if the machinery is not available. This lateralised treatment method reactivates parts of the brain that are closed off during trauma, a common coping mechanism. Looking at the machine in front of me, the cynic inside me wondered if this sophisticated machine could really relieve anxiety and pain with literally a flick of the eye.

Anthony asked me to follow the lights back and forth with my eyes for approximately 60–90 seconds. He explained that the emotions and physical sensations surrounding the event were important and we would examine the original events associated with the trauma. He asked me to keep my mind on the event. As my eyes began to flicker from side to side, I began to simultaneously track the lights on the machine. Looking alternately at the left and right panels of the picture, I began to recall the second time I was diagnosed with cancer.

He asked me to see what picture came to mind but said I was not to analyse my thoughts while they were unfolding, as this would interrupt the flow of memories coming forth. This is because analysis is a left brain function, involving the rational part of the brain, whereas memory is related to the functions of the right hemisphere.

Slowly, painfully and vividly, the memories came to mind. My first memory was of the night I gave my son Richard the news that the cancer had returned. That evening he was uncharacter-istically quiet throughout dinner, the atmosphere was heavy but no one commented on the bad news because we all wanted to protect my youngest daughter Julie from the pain of knowing her mum had cancer.

As I began to picture Richard and how he must have felt, a terrible ache consumed me. I remember how he did not take his gaze off me all evening and hardly touched his meal. I knew that by staring at me he was trying to read my mind, wordlessly begging for reassurance that I would be all right. After clearing up the dinner plates, I went upstairs and glanced into his room. He had his back to me, but I could see he was fiddling with stuff on his desk, pretending to be busy. I asked him if he was OK, knowing that he wasn't.

I went over to him and put my arms around him. I wanted to protect him, but I knew he was old enough now to understand. At 18, he rarely liked to show his emotions but he turned round in his chair and put his arms around my waist, resting his head against me. He did not say a word. I stroked his hair and the realisation struck me that he loved me with all his being. I will remember that moment, when my boundless love for him was reflected back, until my dying day.

Anthony asked me on a scale of zero to 10 how I rated the feeling brought on by the memory, zero being good and 10 being stressful. I answered eight. As I recalled the evening, I remembered my words of reassurance to him. 'Listen, Rich, you know I'm a fighter. You know I am not going to let this thing take me down.'

'I know, Mum,' he had replied. He was trying so hard not to break down in front of me, yet he caught my mood exactly. He knew that I would do what I could to help myself. But my heart ached for him, this boy who was not quite a man. His world was falling apart and his only thoughts were that his mother was going to die. I felt so guilty, so responsible – thinking, dear God, what have I done to give myself this cancer and take me away from my children who need me so much?

At this point in the session, tears were pouring down my face, it was not a vague recollection of this past life episode, but an intense visual sensation that stemmed from this distressing experience. Anthony explained that these altruistic feelings were natural for a mother. Mothers often feel a tremendous amount of guilt and assume personal responsibility for the pain that life presents to their children. But these dark thoughts of self-blame can colour your perception.

He asked me to picture us a few years into the future and visualise both of us looking at my books and the thousands of people who had been helped by them. Then he repeated his question, asking me where on the scale the feeling was now. I reported it lowering down the scale as he repeated the process. Next he asked me to visualise one of my seminars. That was easy – I could see myself talking and demonstrating recipes. Richard had helped on many occasions and I imagined him watching me in the background. People were asking him questions and he replied with confidence. Somehow creating a positive picture began to help me replace those hurtful memories.

Anthony continued processing the information until it became less and less disturbing and, eventually, the emotional charge of the memory dropped to zero. As soon as I achieved a peaceful resolution to the memory, he stopped the light machine. In order to completely desensitise the original traumatic event, he asked me to stay in the moment and see if there were any other emotions that came up from that time.

I could not believe the quagmire of emotions that unfolded, feelings that had been dormant for so long.

I could see a very clear, distinct picture of my daughter Sarah holding my hair while I was vomiting just after the chemotherapy treatment had started. I had been vomiting all through the night and into following morning. I had vomited and vomited, until I thought I could vomit no more, and still it went on. Sarah came into the bathroom at one point.

'Mum! You look awful. What can I do?' she had said as she came over and held my hair back while I retched. She had knelt beside me in the bathroom and stroked my hair. 'How are you going to make it through another six months of this?'

Ger had asked me that same question the night before. I hated to see Sarah so worried and frightened, and to know that I was the cause of her pain.

Anthony asked me to make the picture that I was visualising smaller, about the size of the screen on a mobile phone. I tried but my mind began to wander back to Sarah. I remembered telling her how much I would need her help with Julie. 'She needs to be a normal little girl living a normal life,' I had explained through gritted teeth. Before I left the hospital, I was given a bone scan to ascertain whether the cancerous cells had reached my bone marrow. A fairly routine procedure, but the radiographer explained the scan would leave me radioactive for a day or so. She asked me not go near any children or anyone who was pregnant for 24 hours.

This was all I needed – how do you explain that to a five-year-old? It seemed to add insult to injury but I was so thankful to be able to rely on Sarah's help with Julie. Anthony pulled me back to the task in hand, he asked that I refocus my vision of the event in black and white. As I began to linger over the image I had created in my mind's eye, I noticed it fading.

Unfortunately, just as I began to erase one overwhelming pang another one came to mind. It was a picture of Julie distraught and confused.

'Are you sick, Mama?' she asked. I could see she was frightened.

'Yes, a little,' I managed to stammer. 'Don't you worry, I'll be better later.' I edged away from her, anxious not to zap her with my radioactive body, but she lingered, reluctant to leave me. I knew she wanted a hug – she hated seeing me ill.

'Can I sit on your lap?'

'Not until tomorrow. We'll have lots of cuddles then.' She turned away unhappily. My poor little mite, all she wanted was to be cuddled and comforted and to be told everything was going to be all right. What she needed more than anything was the very thing I had been forbidden to give her.

Anthony's voice roused me from this distressing memory.

He directed me to now relive the experience with Julie. I tried hard to concentrate in the hope of replacing these negative thoughts with positive feelings but the pain and intensity of the emotions that accompanied these memories were beyond words. I remembered the following day how she shut herself in her bedroom and would not let Sarah in. As I went in, she was picking up beads and replacing them in a basket.

'What's wrong, love?' I asked as I cupped her sweet, trusting face in my hands. She said nothing, and just shook her head. 'Come on, you can tell me. What is it?'

'I don't know,' came a very small voice. She burst into tears. I sat on her bed and gathered her into my arms. She lay on me and cried and cried. I held her while her small body was wracked with sobs, her tears soaking into my shirt.

'It's OK, everything will be fine, don't worry,' I murmured repeatedly, kissing her head, smoothing her tears away with my fingertips until gradually her sobs subsided.

My little pet, still only a baby, was having to deal with all this, no matter how hard we had tried to protect her, we could not keep all of it away from her.

Although I still felt the same emotional charge as I played out these scenes in my mind, Anthony carried on reconstructing and regenerating the mental images until the remaining feelings no longer felt upsetting. He asked me to give Julie the benefit of hindsight.

This would give her the opportunity to view the event after it had occurred. As I tried to create a different picture, I imagined my little girl looking at me as I am today, alive and well, knowing that many years in the future I would still be there to take care of her. As this image came to mind, I could see how she gained strength from this, how it lifted her mood and she began to smile. As the sequence of events began to fade, I heaved a sigh of relief.

There is no denying that love and fear are two of our strongest emotions but as I began to release the emotional charge of these events, I began to see them from a more detached perspective. Anthony helped me work through the disturbing memories that I associated with that time until they became linked with a positive belief.

I felt such relief in reframing these events in a healthier light. What lesson did I draw from this major release of those painful memories? Cognitive reorganising communicates on multiple levels of awareness and enables negative, painful emotions to give way to more resolved, empowered feelings. Anthony explained that we consistently need outlets for emotional expression and this is a healthy pathway for getting in touch with our feelings.

Others who have experienced this type of psychotherapy have told me they believe it is a valid avenue for consideration when you are trying to access deep emotional blockages and remove layers of conditioning that restrict lifestyle choices. My belief is that this therapy is a vehicle to enlightenment, development and healing.

Chapter Nine

Medicine for the Soul

'Into each life some rain must fall.'

HENRY WADSWORTH LONGFELLOW

Surprisingly when death stalks us through a physical crisis, it can highlight the need for fulfilment in other aspects of our lives. Time and time again when people share the trials and tribulations of their gruelling journeys, I have found that these have been the catalysts for change on emotional, mental and spiritual levels.

Crisis can be transforming, Fritjof Capra wrote about 'the profound connection between crisis and change'. He referred to the term the Chinese use for 'crisis' – *wei-ji* – the word is composed of the characters for 'danger' and 'opportunity'. For many, that is exactly what crisis turns out to be, a great opportunity for personal growth.

One woman, who had been swept along the road of this arduous journey, explained that her challenge with cancer had propelled her to focus on areas of her life that she had previously neglected.

She had spent decades trying to keep everything going and, because she had been preoccupied with addressing life's challenges, she had ignored a deeper need for spiritual growth.

Carl Jung, the Swiss psychologist, cautioned that modern society relies too heavily on science and logic and that people would benefit from integrating spirituality into their lives. Jung, a visionary of his time, felt it was real-life experience that really counted. I myself believe that spirituality is integrated into our daily actions and develops from our everyday experiences.

Running through the core of this development is love, forgiveness and acceptance. These three areas are fundamental to spiritual development and characterise human spirituality. Accepting ourselves for who we are and where we are in life and not where we want to be is essential in this progression. Body and mind function correctly when we reconnect with our inner selves. Jung also emphasised that every person had a unique story to tell.

Maureen's Story

Maureen was a down-to-earth woman who had real charisma, even though she was not aware of it. She had taken a few knocks in her life, including the death of her treasured husband Ian, some 15 years before I met her. When Ian had died suddenly of a heart attack, it had been a devastating blow that Maureen had found painful, she had ached with grief. Not a day went by that she did not think of her beloved Ian, who had been her soul mate. Maureen had set aside a space in her heart for Ian and the void his death had created would always be there.

On top of the difficulties of mending her broken heart and moving on after her major loss, she was now the sole custodian of their two young children, Shay who was five and Louise who was three at the time. She modestly described herself as a less than perfect mother, which was not what I saw, in fact she was a devoted mother who had a tireless dedication and commitment to her family. She was a wonderful role model to her children during their formative years. Her abounding love, untiring sacrifice and selfless giving set such an example to her son and daughter. They were all she had and she would have given them the sun, the moon and the stars if she could.

However, a better future seemed like an impossible dream because Maureen faced financial disaster. A few years before his death, Ian's small business, which had been in trouble for some time had failed. He had faced one problem after another throughout that time and had been under enormous strain. He had tried to act like he was in control, and taking it all in his stride, but Maureen was convinced that it was the strain and pressure cause by his business collapsing that had led to his heart attack. Apart from her inadequate widow's pension, Maureen had no money.

It wasn't easy, she worked hard and earned little money, they lived a meagre existence, there were no luxuries. Back then, work was scarce but Maureen found a job as a cleaner with several women who needed someone to do light housework – though there was nothing light about it and she cooked, cleaned and washed five days a week for years. There were days she was so exhausted, she thought she would drop. When things got the better of her, Maureen would cry herself to sleep, hoping she would wake up to find Ian taking care of them.

After numerous years of trying to make ends meet, the upkeep of her role as single parent proved too much for Maureen, as she became weighed down with the responsibilities of work and family. Holding everything together for the family eventually took its toll on her health.

When the bombshell came, she never imagined she had such strength within herself. After two or three weeks of in-depth tests and consultations, Maureen's consultant made clear the severity of her situation. Advanced malignant neoplasm of the pancreas.

She told me there was an eerie stillness in the room as her doctor spoke and something in his grave expression made her realise something was terribly wrong. She looked at this kind, straight-talking man and wondered how she would phrase the question. She needed a straight answer. 'How long?' she managed to ask.

He looked up and she saw a flash of distress cross his face. There was a pause, his brow furrowed then he looked her in the eye. 'About three months,' he said confidently, as if it was something he had said many times before and would say many times in the future. He explained that this was the best case scenario; it was an automatic death sentence. The cancer was so widespread that no medical treatment was offered.

Now labelled untreatable and terminal, Maureen struggled to hide her emotions as he explained there was very little that could be done for her at this stage. The words spun round in her head, she felt flayed alive. In the blink of an eye, her life came crashing down around her, she was face to face with death.

As her doctor reassured her they would do everything they could to make her comfortable, the shock and disbelief really began to sink in. She had an overwhelming feeling of doom as she realised her life was drawing to a close.

In the past, I have witnessed case after case where people felt they were condemned after receiving such a diagnosis; it's a very vulnerable time. The doctors words become engrained in their minds and these words can trigger old beliefs about what cancer means.

When you are told you have cancer, the psychological impact is massive. Often feelings of fear, hopelessness and helplessness set in and you may feel you have lost control. Many of these sufferers have difficulty controlling the spiral of worries that comes after they receive a verdict like this and they go downhill rapidly.

In the aftermath of such a diagnosis, you need a level of control to help you harness the healing process. A fatalistic response can profoundly limit your options, as it interferes with your ability to respond to the diagnosis in a positive and beneficial way. When hope is taken away, so is the future, and an inevitable slow progression of diminishing health follows, for those who accept their fate.

This was not Maureen. She was not about to give up and accept the dreadful fate she had been given. Although she was raw with shock, barely able to see the road through her tears, she pulled herself together sufficiently to drive home. An hour later, she was standing in my living room.

I noticed the pallor in her face and my sense that something was desperately wrong was confirmed when she collapsed onto the sofa. My heart sank, I looked at her questioning, instantly on my guard. 'How bad is it?' I asked delicately.

With great effort she explained that the doctor's words had been 'about three months'.

She managed a rueful smile. 'I swear to God, if I am going down, I am going down fighting. I am not on my way to the undertaker yet, I going to pray for some new scientific discovery – some new drug,' she declared bravely.

This desire for a magic bullet is by no means unique to Maureen, it resonates with many of the people I help. The search for one therapy that will help them recover, whether it is the latest vitamin pill or a new scientifically proven drug, is in my experience hard to pin down. I have seen people take all manner of alternative treatments and concoctions in the hope that this will be the *one treatment* that will heal them. Equally, I have experienced first hand and seen many others suffer dramatic side effects of medical treatments and pharmaceutical drugs. A complete recovery of physical and emotional health comes from good food, an active lifestyle and a good mental outlook.

I asked if she would seek a second opinion but Maureen came from a generation who did not ask questions and she had an unquestioning faith in her doctor.

Throughout the dark days that followed, Maureen had bouts of panic. The feeling of impotent fury began to show. She became overwhelmed with anger, fear and anxiety and her mind was a mass of conflicting emotions. She was desperately trying to hang on to normality but her mental anguish and concerns for her son and daughter deeply disturbed her. She was full of sadness not so much for herself, as for them. How on earth was she going to drop this bombshell on them? She had loved them with all her being from the moment they were conceived, they were so special to her; it was overwhelming. Now she wanted to protect them from all this. She prayed to God to shield them from the pain and sorrow she feared lay ahead.

Maureen felt truly isolated as people spoke in hushed tones around her and looked at her with pitying glances, keeping their distance and not knowing what to say. Cancer can be hard to talk about; it seems such a taboo subject that it inspires fear and silence in people. I can't understand how those Maureen knew could have been so oblivious to her pain, but they could not have known how alone she felt. She felt marked out as different and tragic, and this estrangement only made her feel more isolated. She had never needed comfort and closeness more, yet she had never felt so cut off from normal human contact.

I remember thinking how fortunate I was when word spread around my village that I was ill, I was inundated with visitors, neighbours and friends they called non-stop to see how I was doing, it was a real blessing at the time. As Maureen watched others carry out their daily tasks absorbed in their own worlds and completely unaware of the turmoil she was feeling, she wondered why she had been singled out for destruction.

She had done her best throughout life to stay on the straight and narrow. All she had ever wanted was to raise her family, now she was torturing herself, wondering if she could have prevented her illness.

As I sat in silence and listened, I searched for the words to comfort her. Although I was filled with empathy for her, I could not find the right words to make her feel better, so I just listened. The one thing she knew she could definitely do was pray, and she prayed then as never before.

As Maureen tried to cling to hope and gain some order and certainty in her life, she read every book she could get her hands on. There was an edge of desperation about her as she trawled through impossible amounts of information. She felt totally bombarded by her findings, there were so many 'experts' out there. At her wits' end, and unsure of where to turn to next, she feared her time was slipping away. She almost reached breaking point when she came across the Simonton Cancer Center.

Maureen had a gut feeling about their treatment and prevention approach to treating disease. I encouraged her to go with her gut instincts. Learning to trust your gut can be a valuable tool when it comes to health – as nobody knows your body better than you. For far too long, this sixth sense has been marginalised and forgotten in Western thinking. Trusting your instincts can help you move beyond the dilemma of needing to find logical reasons for every situation. We often argue against our unconscious guidance with rational thinking. When this happens, important intuitive messages are ignored and disregarded by logical thoughts. Niggling feelings of doubt often stand in the way of instinctual decisions because we have not learned to trust our intuition.

Maureen's face lit up for a brief moment before darkening. 'I have to do it now – I can't put it off,' she said courageously.

I marvelled at her bravery and determination.

Although Maureen had set her mind on going to the centre in California, she could not afford the expensive trip. She had some savings but they fell short of the amount she needed.

The hope Maureen had of gaining peace of mind immediately sparked me into action and, for a time, raising money for her trip became a key focus in my life. Before I knew it, we had raised the necessary money and she headed off to America. It was a wise choice. Enrolled in Simonton's programme, Maureen found the calm she was looking for. A woman who had grieved inwardly for years, and rarely showed her emotions, she was soon to open up like a flower. Feelings that she internalised for so long unfolded and her sprit soared free.

The Simonton Center

Dr Carl Simonton, a radiation oncologist took a psychological approach to treating disease. Simonton is widely praised and rightfully so, because of his pioneering work in the field of mind–body medicine. He devoted his life to researching the psychological impact of thoughts, beliefs, feelings and mental attitudes on his patients' health. He and his wife Stephanie co-founded The Simonton Research Center and they are recognised worldwide as leaders in their field. Dr Simonton won a Humanitarian Award from the Cancer Control Society in recognition for his 30 years of ground-breaking work in the field of oncology.

Simonton's unique approach addresses the fundamental link between emotional states, stress, negative thoughts and physical well-being. It was the first systematic, emotional intervention used in the treatment of cancer. This total approach to fighting cancer combines traditional medical management with emotional and psychological support for both the cancer patient and their chosen support person (friend or family member) to create the most favourable environment for recovery.

Their approach is based on the belief that our state of mind can influence our ability to survive any disease and improve our quality of health. The results they have achieved have been remarkable; Simonton's patients have a survival rate twice the American national norm and, in many cases, have experienced dramatic remissions or total cures. Their programme became known as the Simonton Approach and, in 1973, it was approved by the Surgeon General's Office, gaining both national and international attention. His beliefs have been accepted by mainstream medicine.

Most of the people at the centre had received diagnoses from their doctors saying that they were 'medically incurable'. Carl Simonton became intent on finding out why some patients died while others recovered their health, despite the fact that the diagnosis and treatment was the same for both. He found that those who recovered (most of whom had little expectation of seeing their next follow-up appointment) had something in common.

These unusual achievers believed they were able to exert some influence over the course of their disease. He also found that they had a strong will to live. Simonton believed that if the patient actively participates in their recovery, they may well exceed their life expectancy and significantly alter the quality of their life.

An important concept in psychology, which helps to explain this, is 'locus of control'. Developed in 1954 by Julian Rotter as a key aspect of personality, it refers to whether or not a person believes that control over events in their lives lies inside or outside of them, whether it is internal or external. People who feel they don't have control over the events in their lives tend to have an external locus of control; these people believe that some higher power or fate controls their life. Those with an internal locus of control believe that they control themselves and their life. As M. E. P. Seligman wrote in *Helplessness: On Depression, Development and Death*: 'This feeling of being in control of one's own destiny is important as a series of negative events can lead to "learned helplessness".'

When we face health challenges, our natural reaction is one of fear, and our thoughts tend to focus on what we don't want, rather than focusing on returning to a state of health and wholeness. By becoming more aware of our thought processes, we can change them from negative to positive, when this happens the patient becomes the locus of control.

For decades, the psychological aspect of cancer has been largely ignored, the emotional needs of people with the disease are left untreated as the focus is on treating the physical disease. Psychological support during this major period of distress is essential. When such interventions are tailored and adapted to suit the needs of the patient, through appropriate education and support, the majority of people find the mental impact they have been experiencing is reduced and they are able to cope and adjust.

Carl Simonton came to understand that thoughts, beliefs, feelings and mental attitudes were all important factors that affect health. He taught techniques such as visual imagery, physical exercise, relaxation and goal setting. Simonton found that these techniques helped his patients to harness the progression of their illness and that it assisted in their recovery. He taught his patients how to cultivate and integrate these processes into their daily routine. Focusing on the healing process develops that all-important *survivor's mindset*. For those who participate in such a life-altering programme, the value is it puts the theories into practise.

Of course, Carl Simonton realised that as with anything in life, there are no guarantees but those teaching his techniques do not give false hope to the people who flock to the centre in California. They believe that if a patient is given reasonable expectation of survival, there chances of recovery can be increased through the work done at the centre.

Believe me, in these situations, pessimistic thoughts turn into barriers and advice turns into salvation. Remember, hope is an important element for the cancer patient; it can enhance recovery just as the absence of hope can inhibit it. I have seen personally how it influenced my ability to get involved in my own recovery. When you take an active role in your health by tapping into mental and physical resources, you can work in conjunction with harmless medical treatments to increase your chances of recovery.

Thanks to Simonton's pioneering work and that of many others in the field of psycho-oncology, this issue is being addressed and the message is now beginning to spread throughout the world.

Maureen's Inner Transformation

Somehow, Maureen's endeavours to find a peaceful end to her life brought her meaning and fulfilment. Her inner transformation came from her desperate need for peace and understanding. This understanding gave her an inner strength that helped her face the realities of her situation. She seemed to rise above the limitations of her physical condition to fulfil such a deep need within herself that it helped ease her way through her struggle to come to terms with the fact that her life was drawing to a close.

As she worked her way towards this understanding, the hidden depths of her existence provided a ray of light at the end of the tunnel and she found a true appreciation of her achievements in her memorable life.

Her rising consciousness illuminated the way forward into her spirit. As a new dawn of spiritual consciousness broke, she dealt with her fears and went through to the other side.

Abraham Maslow, a crusader for humanistic psychology, wrote extensively about this phenomenon. His main contribution was theoretical work in the field of motivation of human needs. He presented his famous 'hierarchy of needs' within the frame of a pyramid. Maslow contended that as humans have evolved, they have developed a number of needs that are arranged in order of their innate power. At the peak of his pyramid sits self-actualisation. This is where the individual becomes aware of his or her own full potential. Maslow presented this actualising tendency as the person's desire to grow and develop a deeper understanding of peace and self-fulfilment. He theorised that people who reach self-actualisation sometimes experience a state of transcendence.

I witnessed such a change in Maureen after her trip to the Simonton Center. Although she went through a steep learning curve, she found a profound sense of peace far beyond anything she had known. This enriching experience gave Maureen a fresh way of relating to herself and her life. The centre may have taught her the techniques of visualisation and relaxation, but Maureen learned – as I and so many others have learned too – that peace comes from within. She learned to live fully in the moment.

The trip to the Simonton Center prepared her admirably for the path that lay ahead. On her return, I noticed a shift in how she perceived her situation. Maureen had become calmer and more serene, her smile and cheerfulness had returned, she had a sort of radiance about her, a light that burned brightly from within. What stands out in my mind is that, despite her physical weakness, her unconstrained personality developed towards a healthy state of mind. She could have withdrawn into a silent black hole. Instead, she found freedom in her need for knowledge and understanding. By fulfilling that need she moved to the next level of self-actualisation. No longer imprisoned within fear and despair, she found a profound joy and meaning to her life

I cannot rationalise the altered state of consciousness Maureen discovered, it was as if she had found a treasure, a powerful force that made her more accepting of what was going to happen. Perhaps it was a connection with the divine or a piece of heaven here on earth. Whatever it was, Maureen was a changed woman who was now unbelievably content and at peace with the world.

What at first had seemed like a tragedy, for her turned out to be a deep enlightenment of a kind that many people never experience.

I know we can only theorise or speak from personal experience but I questioned if the average person could gain insight into the true meaning of spirituality and human existence if they have not witnessed or experienced that state of consciousness. Are these mysterious and largely uncharted depths of consciousness only available to a small minority of people like Maureen who look into the abyss?

We discussed in depth how when you reach this particular stage in life, you somehow access a part of your mind that is more attuned, it is a different world that in some way gives a rare glimpse of life in the spiritual domain.

'Experiencing every day as a blessing, freed me from the mountainous shadow that was crowding in around me,' Maureen said, speaking calmly and soothingly. 'Confronting death made me see the beauty of human life, the great job I made of raising my beautiful children who I am so proud of.'

To others, Maureen appeared to be dying; to me she appeared so alive. While this thin, wasted soul still yearned for the invigorating energy of life, the process of self-discovery enabled Maureen to live in the moment, as the moment was all that she was sure of. She explained to me how her senses had become overwhelmingly powerful – her sight, touch and smell had all become acute.

We chatted about how these life-altering events affect the senses. Curiously, when you engage fully with the senses, everything you see, everything you touch, becomes loaded with meaning. She explained how her previously untapped sense of smell had heightened dramatically. That is because smell is one of our most immediate senses, nasal sensory receptors are closely linked to memory and directly activate and affect the limbic system, an interior part of the brain that is associated with emotions. Maureen's biggest regret was that she had not spent more time taking care of herself and less time working.

I had such a connection with her that devoting my time to her awoke within me a side of my being that I hadn't really known existed; I somehow became more connected, more compassionate. Maureen was one of those rare and special people you meet in your life.

On the night she died, I had an overwhelming dream about her, in which she walked towards me smiling. She seemed younger and more vibrant. I recall a feeling of relief that she was well and healthy. I could clearly see she was happy, as she looked at me with a tender expression. She reached for my right hand, gently gave it a little squeeze we bade our final farewells and she walked off into the distance. Her smile conveyed to me that her quest for physical health was over. At last she was liberated from the constraints of her physical condition and now she was happy to be moving on.

In ancient times, dreaming was considered to be communication with the divine. In recent times, scientists have come to believe that dreams are the way the unconscious mind relays messages to the conscious mind. The overall significance of dreams may at first appear of no consequence but they should not be discounted just because we lack the understanding to interpret their meaning. I am no expert at unravelling the meaning of dreams, but I believe they give a clue to what is going on in the subconscious mind.

When I woke the next morning I told Ger about my dream, saying, 'I am sure Maureen has passed away.'

He instantly dismissed it as 'just a dream'.

Later that day, Maureen's daughter rang me to tell me her mother had passed on during the night. I talked to her about my beautiful dream and she found great comfort in the mystery and wonder of it. Prior to this event, I had never experienced anything as profoundly vivid and real in a dream. I know at the time I had a deep affinity with Maureen's plight, but it was a spiritual experience to feel so connected with her life.

Although Maureen did not have the luxury of time and cruelly lost her battle for life, against all the odds, she found that in every hardship there lies a blessing.

Maureen came face to face with the end of her journey and as terrible as it was, I was not saddened by her death. I had witnessed such a personal transformation, extraordinary peace, a calmness that replaced dialogue and a strength of character that I felt compelled to share her experience so that others might benefit.

Chapter Ten

The Forgotten Hero

All power is from within, and is absolutely under your control;
it comes through exact knowledge and by the voluntary exercises
of exact principles.'

CHARLES F. HAANEL

O ur greatest defence against disease is our immune system –
it is nature's wonderful self-healing mechanism. It is our
immune system that comes to our rescue when we are sick. This
important fact is all too often overlooked when it comes to
healing. The body's natural defences help us heal cuts, bruises and
broken bones and they can also help us overcome more serious
conditions.

This in-built safety feature keeps a close watch for foreign
invaders, and attacks and destroys anything threatening that enters
the body; its only objective is our survival.

Without the immune system, the door is wide open to bacteria,
viruses, parasites and toxins to invade our bodies. When we die,
these organisms begin to engulf our bodies within hours, proving

how powerful this intricate system is at protecting us from attack while we are alive. Yet all too often, the immune system appears to be the forgotten hero in protecting our health.

Many of the symptoms that we associate with illness are, in fact, our body's attempts to regain a state of health. As it attempts to elicit an immune response, the symptoms of fever, inflammation, coughing and sneezing are all signs that the immune system is working efficiently. This is a crucial point to remember, otherwise we may suppress the symptoms of illness and hamper the healing process by not allowing nature to carry out its work.

John Beard, Professor of Comparative Embryology at the Edinburgh University Medical School, showed that cancer is a healing mechanism as early as 1904 and was one of the first doctors to make this connection.

Many years later, in his book *Cancer is not a Disease – It's a Survival Mechanism*, Andreas Moritz explained that cancer is more a healing response than it is a disease. 'The disease is the body's attempt to cure itself of an existing imbalance, a desperate attempt by the body to stay alive.'

He believes that during serious illness, the body is not trying to kill you, as its original genetic design always favours the preservation of life and would not permit self-destruction. He wrote that:

> *Cancer cells, like all other cells, know that if the body dies, they will die as well. A cancerous tumor is neither the cause of progressive destruction nor does it actually lead to the death of the body. The drastic reduction or shut down of vital nutrients*

190

supplies to the cells of an organ is not primarily a consequence
of a cancerous tumor, but actually its biggest cause.

Moritz proposes that cancer will only occur after all other defence
or healing mechanisms in the body have failed. He provides
evidence that people who suffer with cancer would most likely die
quickly unless they actually grew cancer cells, and that cancer is
indeed part of the body's complex survival responses. He says that:

Like every other disease it is but a toxicity crisis, it marks the
body's final attempt to rid itself of septic poisons and acidic
compounds accumulated because the body was not able to
properly remove metabolic waste, toxins and decomposing cells.
The consequence of waste build-up in the cell environment is
that cancer cells not only become deprived of oxygen and other
vital nutrients, but also begin to suffocate in their own waste.
Out of necessity the genes generated a new blueprint that
enabled them to survive without oxygen and instead use some
of the metabolic waste products for energy. Cancer is never the
cause of a disease but rather a reaction to a far-advanced,
unhealthy physical condition.

While many of us may struggle to understand this concept of
healing as a solution to the cancer problem, seeing disease as part
of the body's preservation response throws a different light on
many of today's methods of healing, and certainly challenges
mainstream beliefs.

Moritz believes that we need to learn the skills of healing ourselves
and states that:

Every person with a sound medical background knows that the symptom of an illness is not the real illness, yet the majority of doctors today treat the symptom as if it were the disease. This symptom-orientated approach to treating disease generates a tremendous number of potential symptomatic side effects that in turn require further treatments. Since none of the chosen treatment modalities are symptom-orientated, there are bound to be continuously escalating complications. This trend will continue only for as long as the masses remain ignorant of their potential self-healing abilities.

Defence Mechanisms

During our evolutionary history, the human body developed a series of strategic mechanisms necessary to keep us alive and in good health. Our body is exposed daily to millions of micro-organisms that cause diseases. The most common micro-organisms with which we are constantly in contact are viruses, bacteria and fungi, and we come into contact with them through touching, breathing, and through our eyes and mouth.

Some mechanisms specialise in stopping toxins produced by micro-organisms from spreading throughout the body. Others are more direct; they repair injuries caused by bumps, cuts, ultraviolet light, chemicals and burns. There are also other important mechanisms of defence that specialise in eliminating cancerous cells from the body. These mechanisms depend on the skin, mucus membranes, chemicals, fever and inflammation to resist the micro-organism invasion. The body also creates specialised defence cells to combat those micro-organisms more directly.

There are many familiar healing responses that we often misinterpret as illness, such as fever, which is an attempt to inhibit the growth of some micro-organisms by elevating the body temperature. Inflammation helps to eliminate toxins generated by micro-organisms and carry the remaining foreign materials away from the site of injury and prevent them from spreading to other organs of the body. Coughing and sneezing are reactions that help to accelerate the movement of mucus and eliminate the foreign substance of micro-organisms.

There are several other components of the immune system that mount attacks on organisms that breach its barriers, but it would take a whole book to fully explain the extraordinary features of this forgotten hero. Of course, there are multitudes of ways that people get sick. Immunodeficiency diseases are areas of intense scientific study but the bottom line is that the elaborate and dynamic network of these in-built healing forces can restore well-being if we give it the correct ammunition and back-up to mount its attacks.

This is no surprise to the countless people who have recovered from life-threatening illnesses.

You may wonder why so many of us have become so susceptible to disease – what makes the immune system so weak that it loses its ability to protect itself? Our modern way of life has contributed enormously to making us less resilient to disease. High-stress lifestyles, junk food, and other poor-quality food that are laden with pesticides, toxins and pollutants, chlorinated and fluoridated water, and electromagnetic radiation are all causes of disease. These damaging lifestyle elements interfere with the harmonious functioning of the body and can wipe out or slow down the normal functions of the immune system.

Many of them, such as fluoride, are known poisons that help to advance opportunistic diseases such as cancer and enable them to become impostors in our bodies. Obviously, if we are to reverse this situation and prepare the ground for a healthy immune system, it makes perfect sense to eliminate them. You cannot make your body healthy if you have a depleted, worn out immune system, but if you correct the underlying causes of disease, you can exploit the weaknesses of that disease. Subsequently, the odds are stacked in your favour of winning the fight against that particular illness.

Immune-Boosting Therapies

Oxygen Therapy

Today we can utilise some of the most advanced technology in the treatment of diseases such as cancer, yet as far back as 1931, the bio-chemist Otto Warburg established that oxygen is an essential element for fighting cancer. Many others within the scientific community have verified his findings most notably the molecular biologist Dr Stephen Levine, who states that, 'Lack of oxygen in the tissues is the fundamental cause of all degenerative diseases.'

Warburg won a Nobel Prize in 1931 for his discovery of this link between insufficient oxygen and cancer. He found cancer cells need a low-oxygen environment to survive. Hypoxia (low-oxygen levels) is linked to a range of diseases from arthritis, bowel disease and cancer. Lack of oxygen leads to stagnation in tissues, and this actively encourages the growth of cancer tumours.

Dr Warburg stated:

> 'Nobody today can say that one does not know what cancer and its prime cause are. On the contrary, there is no disease whose prime cause is better known, so that today ignorance is no longer an excuse that one cannot do more about prevention. That prevention of cancer will come there is no doubt, for man wishes to survive.

One hope in the treatment to prevent disease is the use of high-pressure oxygen chambers; this is known as hyperbaric oxygen therapy. This therapy is an effective way of oxygenating the areas of the body that are deprived of oxygen. Often used in the treatment of Caisson disease (otherwise known as 'diver's disease' or 'the bends'). Decompression sickness is suffered by a person exposed to a decrease in pressure in their body. If a diver ascends too quickly from a dive, oxygen therapy is used to adapt the body to the atmospheric pressure.

Breathing in pure oxygen by nasal canula in a pressurised chamber pushes oxygen into the cells that are starved of this vital element. High saturation of oxygen delivered by this type of therapy penetrates deep into tissues, organs, muscles, bones and the nervous system. When pure oxygen is pumped into the blood stream, healing is directed into the body to speed recovery. Because it stimulates the immune system, oxygen boosts the number of immune protecting t-cells. Oxygen levels drop as we age and this causes stagnation in the blood vessels. Hyperbaric oxygen therapy is a recognised treatment in the UK's national health service.

Warburg concluded that oxygenating the cells was the best way to fight cancer, viruses, bacteria and infections.

Far Infrared Therapy

Another way to increase the flow of oxygen to the cells is to mildly heat up the body to 37 degrees Celsius. Far infrared heat can penetrate deep into the body to help maintain good health, well-being and prevent disease. Its rays are absorbed deep into the tissues, and this increases circulation and stimulates the flow of blood to the peripheral areas. The molecular vibration of this therapy excites the cells and fastens the metabolic exchanges between the cells. The increased blood flow carries the hyper-oxygenated blood and any vitamins and minerals the blood may be carrying to the areas of the body most in need of healing.

When the body's core temperature is raised slightly, it stimulates the immune system into action. At the cellular level, the increased presence of heat and oxygen enables the metabolic rate and immune system function to be maximised. Infrared heat plus oxygen also make the synovial fluid in joints and disk space healthier, as joints are lubricated and nourished. Far infrared heat relieves tension, pressure and pain. Infrared therapy brings your immune system into balance, enabling your body to function more efficiently.

An Integrated Approach

There are many people who were given only a few weeks to live who have pulled through and conquered cancer when they changed their lifestyles. David Servan-Schreiber was a rising neuroscientist with his own laboratory and funding for brain imaging. During the course of testing new equipment, he discovered a tumour the size of a walnut lodged in his own brain.

In his book, *A New Way of Life*, he tells the story of how, as a researcher and scientist who believed only in conventional treatments, he became an integrative physician who realises the importance and power of the body's natural defences against chronic disease. Servan-Schreiber makes a compelling case for taking part in your own healing, explaining: 'Every day at every meal we can choose the food that will defend our bodies against the invasion of cancer.'

Questions I am asked repeatedly is why it is that the medical profession do not appear to recognise the role of nutrition and complementary therapies in the boosting of the immune system. Why don't they look favourably on these practices as a source of both healing and prevention of disease? Why, indeed, do they focus so little on the prevention of disease in the first place?

These are fair questions that touch on truths that we rarely acknowledge. I also find this puzzling, but perhaps it is because medical treatments are based solely on pharmacology. Whether this blinkered approach is simply short-sighted or whether it happens because only the treatments tested by double blind trials are taken seriously is up for debate, maybe it's a bit of both. Either way, I have found no clear answers to these questions. Many patients try to define these questions and find answers to them in their quest for recovery.

What I have found is an overwhelming consensus amongst patients for a need to have an integrated approach.

If only traditional Western medicine and complementary therapists could join forces and talk openly about ways of fixing these problems, then maybe we could halt the massive deterioration and spread of the endless list of modern diseases. A development such as this could be the gateway to ending some of the world's most dreaded diseases and finally solving this ongoing problem, once and for all. Are we not more likely to hit on what works best to correct these conditions if we have an eclectic approach? One of the greatest defects of modern medicine is that it neglects to tap into the healing mechanisms of the mind and body.

However, studies in the past seven years, in both the UK and the USA now show that 40 per cent of people use alternative medicine before they visit their GP, that situation may well be changing. I wonder if Hippocrates, the father of medicine, was alive today, would he be leading the way in pharmacology or complimentary therapies? On the surface, they may appear to be different ends of the spectrum but surely their objective is the same, to return the patient to health. I suspect Hippocrates might try to bridge the gap and seek a balance between both.

Traditional Chinese Medicine

As we have seen, the immune system is our in-built safety mechanism against disease, so what are the best ways to strengthen it? If we look at Eastern medicine, we can see how it uses methods of increasing resistance to disease through boosting the immune system. Traditional Chinese medicine has used the approach of activating the immune system's defence mechanism for over 4,000 years. The Chinese do not subscribe to the idea of suppressing physical symptoms.

In fact, Eastern medicine is based on observing a complete picture of the patient's behavioural patterns. Treating the body as a whole rather than just individual, symptomatic parts can give an in-depth analysis of the underlying cause of illness and disease.

When assessing a patient, emotional issues, eating habits, work and exercise are all taken into account. The practitioner will hone in on important clues, with questions such as: When did it start? Has it happened before? What have you done about it so far? Looking at the impact of the patient's lifestyle can provide valuable clues for the practitioner. Seeing the patient's life in a broad context helps the practitioner direct treatment towards the underlying cause of the problem. A tailor-made plan of acupuncture, dietary changes, medicinal teas and herbs is then implemented in order to return the patient to full physical and mental health. This is not a mystical or magical formula but a legitimate approach backed by thousands of years of practical application.

Chinese medicine concentrates primarily on healing, whereas Western medicine concentrates more on treatment and disease management. This is another area that seems to be changing as many Western pharmacologists are now analysing plants, roots and herbs because they are known to be less toxic than chemical drugs. From nature's vast herbal pharmacopoeia, the practitioner selects combinations of herbs, each one of which has a specific purpose, and they are then prescribed specifically to suit the needs of the individual patient. The practitioner monitors the patient's progress closely and alters and reduces the prescriptions doses accordingly.

The traditional Chinese approach is safer and more cost effective than the intensive interventions of modern technologically based medicine. Furthermore, consider the vast number of Chinese people using this approach to great effect. The collective wisdom of their healing traditions is widely recognised as one of their greatest assets. Traditional Chinese medicine is recognised by the World Health Organization. It is no longer solely the preserve of the Chinese people, as it is now becoming more accessible to all of us with many Chinese practices now established in most Western cities and towns.

Elaine's story

Today an alarming number of people suffer with irritable bowel syndrome (IBS), a disorder that now affects 10–20 per cent of people in the West. It is notoriously difficult to treat with conventional treatments. Of course as this is a digestive disorder, the Western diet goes a long way towards producing the problem.

Elaine suffered with IBS for years. She had attended two different specialists and had an array of medical interventions, x-rays, colonoscopy, barium-meal tests and, of course, a variety of drugs. 'Enough to start a pharmacy,' she explained. Her doctors had been treating her symptoms with prescription medications for years, but her condition didn't improve. Her symptoms were not vague digestive problems that she could not pin down, but chronic diarrhoea that she had to battle and deal with daily.

She described herself as a carefree type until this persistent problem came along and affected her family, work and social life. As IBS is often stress related, I asked Elaine if anything had changed in her life since the problem had begun. She explained how since a promotion at work a few years earlier, she had been running around cramming her diary with appointments and meeting deadlines. She admitted she was quite stressed by the various things that cropped up during her hurried day. Weekends were a welcome reprieve from the worries of her working week.

It is not hard to imagine how debilitating the need to have a bowel movement without warning could be. In September 2006, Elaine decided to take a well-earned break when her husband's business took them to China for a two-month period. Naturally enough, this presented a huge problem for Elaine; she was dreading the arduous journey, change of food and the socialising with her husband's business colleagues. Nevertheless, she went on the trip fully armed with a two-month supply of medication.

During the time in China, Elaine's problem returned with a vengeance, and was possibly exacerbated by the change of food. She visited a nearby Chinese doctor recommended by a colleague of her husband and, after a short examination, the doctor told her (through an interpreter) that there was a problem with her colon.

She had given him no information apart from explaining that she had cramps in her stomach. He examined her tongue, ears, eyes, checked different pulses and asked about her diet and lifestyle.

Elaine explained to him that she had had this problem for years and her doctors at home had made many futile attempts to control the problem. The Chinese doctor replied that he did not have much faith in Western medicine because of the toxicity of some of the drugs prescribed. He preferred the tried and tested Chinese medicines, as many of the preparations are non-toxic so they can be used over extended periods of time without damage to the body's systems. He explained that her long-term use of drugs to alleviate her diarrhoea had created a perfect breeding ground for harmful bacteria to multiply, as the friendly bacteria that are needed to populate the gut are often wiped out by drugs.

This made perfect sense to Elaine but she had reservations about the old doctor, believing that he was set in his ways and was not very open-minded. He prescribed acupuncture to stimulate and unblock her body's energy channels, and herbs to sooth and heal the lining of her gut. Amazingly, within two short weeks of receiving the acupuncture and herbs, Elaine's problem subsided. It may not have stood up as a miracle to the medics at home, but this therapeutic intervention was a godsend for Elaine. The trip to China and the old doctor turned out to be a blessing.

The World Health Organization has made it known that there is sufficient medical evidence to prove the effectiveness of acupuncture for the treatment of over 100 conditions. It stimulates the production of endorphins, which act as a natural anaesthetic, relieving pain and strengthening the immune system. Studies have shown that Chinese herbal treatments offer considerable benefit in treating the symptoms of irritable bowel syndrome. In trials independently confirmed by gastroenterologists, bowel symptoms were significantly diminished in patients prescribed the herbal formulations. For people such as Elaine, it strengthens their belief that these therapies are worth a try.

We spend enormous amounts of money and time on research to find treatments and cures for diseases such as arthritis, cancer, heart disease and diabetes. Surely the best strategy would be to explore ways of boosting the immune system and increasing resistance from within, so we don't get these diseases in the first place. The vast majority of us are so entrenched in the thinking and practices of modern medicine that we have forgotten the power of the healing system within.

Chapter Eleven

Thinking Outside the Box

'The best prescription is knowledge.'

DR C. EVERETT KOOP

We have established the power of the mind and body to heal, and that patients who are fully focused and committed to their recovery have, indeed, got a powerful skill set. It can also be said that conflict and friction between mind and body can escalate health problems. As our thoughts produce biological consequences for our physical well-being, then the doctors we trust with our health should be on our wavelength. It dilutes the patient's resolve and therefore their healing power, where a doctor continues to cast doubt on the patient's innate belief systems about well-being.

The best doctor–patient relationship is a partnership; one in which the doctor looks out for the best interests of the patient and does everything he or she can to aid that patient's recovery. A doctor should support the patient's choices for a recovery programme and, if possible, they should work out the recovery plan together. The other important element in this partnership is where the patient takes ownership of their health by making the necessary lifestyle changes to aid recovery – it's a two-way street.

Communication, trust and good management are the cornerstones of the bond between doctor and patient. It plays a vital part in their relationship; understanding the patient's needs hinges on this key skill. Find a doctor that you can relate to, as a stormy, confrontational relationship with your doctor will achieve very little. In the same way as you would source any other service, do some research until you find a health practitioner that resonates with you – someone with whom you can form that vital partnership to assist you on the road to well-being.

The heart of Amy's tale shows how many wonderful doctors have fought to work outside the constraints of conventional medicine.

Initially, Amy did not experience good communication with her doctor. She had just been diagnosed with colon cancer when she contacted me. She was unfortunate in that she had been misdiagnosed and, for quite some time, had been mistakenly treated for Crohn's disease by her family doctor. Over the years, she had taken every medicine her doctor had prescribed for her and while they alleviated the symptoms, none of them gave great results. Then, after a host of tests, the real problem was eventually uncovered.

At that stage, Amy was losing confidence in her doctors, and was starting to suspect that traditional medicine might not hold all the answers. She had left all the decisions about her health to her doctors. However, no longer able to assume they would get it right, she made the decision that she was going to take charge of her recovery. This was her body, so she was no longer willing to go through whatever treatment was meted out to her blindly and acceptingly. She was so disillusioned with the medical team that had been treating her that she had grave doubts about whether or not they had diagnosed her cancer correctly as she found her doctor secretive and evasive in his habit of drip-feeding information to her.

I reasoned with Amy that the doctor probably had her best interests at heart. In his effort to shield her from the truth, he was possibly trying to spare her from the psychological distress of her situation. It is not always helpful for doctors to tell patients their predictions of exactly what lies ahead when they are embarking on one of the toughest periods of their lives.

No one knows how he or she will react to news that they have a life-threatening illness. Each patient reacts differently; some people want to discuss the diagnosis, their fears and the treatment with everyone they meet, while others withdraw into themselves and are unwilling to discuss it at all. These are standard coping strategies following an initial diagnosis.

Some individuals feel threatened when they begin to lose control over their lives, and many cope best with that fear by being included in the decision-making of their treatment plan. The psychological impact of such a serious illness can mean people feel ill-equipped to handle the situation, and they surrender decisions on how to proceed to their medical team. The doctors are left with the difficult decision of how they think a patient will cope.

The diagnosis pretty much tore Amy's life apart and she found it hard to face up to the reality of her situation; she needed time to adjust and gather her thoughts. Even though she did not want to rock the boat and jeopardise her position with the hospital, she was unhappy with the treatment she had received so far. She was determined that, this time, she would take charge and challenge the problem head on. She was going to ask questions, because, after all, this was a serious illness she was dealing with.

Naturally enough, she had concerns about the effectiveness of the treatment and was questioning the infallibility of modern medicine as never before. She described her physician as being a bit distant, with an unapproachable bedside manner. In response to her concerns about the high risk of recurrence within the first two years after surgery, he had baffled her with 'medical jargon'. When she had voiced her apprehension about her treatment, he had brushed her concerns aside, side-stepped the issues and retreated out the door.

Hers were not irrational fears, but real concerns that scared the hell out of her.

As a first step in getting involved in her treatment, she sat down and read the clearly labelled leaflets and labels of the listed possible side effects of her prescription medicines. When she finished chastising herself for having ignored this until now, she became worried about the impact that they might be having on her health. She found it hard to grasp how drugs with devastating side effects could heal her. How could she rest easy when she realised that her immune system would pay a high price because she had used these drugs?

She needed decisive answers to these challenging questions and approached her doctor for assistance in making sense of it. She felt he was irritated by her questions, and his reaction when she asked about nutrition and complementary therapies, was downright hostile. It was clear he would not engage in discussions on the subject. When she pressed him to explain the merits of the treatment he recommended, he insisted it was her only option. She felt that there had to be other doctors with a broader understanding of both conventional and complementary therapies, but she also felt she could not afford to step outside the system.

Many of the doctors and nurses I have taught over the years have had no formal education in nutrition. For some, their intuition tells them that this is a missing link in their treatment methods, and they seek out supplementary knowledge in courses such as the ones I give. This is so important, especially when you consider that every strand of DNA is made from nutrition and every aspect of our body literally and biologically requires nutrition.

Amy was an inquisitive woman who had been brought up in an atmosphere of openness and honesty. It was something her parents were very firm about, impressing upon her that the most important thing was to be truthful. They believed that truth prevails only when both sides are heard, and, in their eyes, this was the foundation of communication. As a result of her upbringing, Amy expected to be given clear information that was open to scrutiny, not indifference that left her distraught and confused. She found that the subject of nutrition was deeply contentious.

Surely nutrition was worth considering since the purpose of eating is to maintain and rebuild the body? But Amy found it difficult to persuade her doctor that food could assist her recovery. After all, she felt it was a reasonable observation that her physical well-being could be improved by what she ate. He told her, 'Nutrition has nothing to do with it.'

In the few books Amy had read on the subject, there appeared to be plenty of credible research on the matter. The US National Cancer Institute of Health linked a range of serious diseases to the foods people eat today. Information from the institute's site claims that:

> *What we eat kills an estimated three out of four Americans each year. Eating a diet that contains 5 to 9 servings of fruits and vegetables a day as part of a healthy, active lifestyle lowers the risk for all of these diseases. Leading causes of death, which include heart disease, high blood pressure, many cancers, diabetes and strokes, are largely preventable through lifestyle choices such as eating more fruits and vegetables. Simple lifestyle changes can save lives and improve your quality of life.*

Amy was in no way dismissing the importance of the medicines and techniques that her doctor had at his disposal. Nor was she trying to replace conventional medicine with alternative therapies. She felt strongly that natural healing therapies could complement her treatment. All she really wanted was a straightforward rounded opinion on what the best options available to her were. She wanted realistic options of the various forms of natural and conventional treatments, because she believed she had a right to choose and participate in a range of treatments. However, she found that she had come up against a brick wall with this particular physician. He was simply not open to the concept of treating the body naturally and his only comment on the nutritional approach was that it was not a viable treatment method because 'the research was weak and hazy about its efficacy'.

Amy felt foolish for daring to ask the questions, and while she was confused about whether there were weaknesses on both sides of the argument, she knew she needed to find out more information on the subject. Her doctor advised her to start treatment immediately and recommended that she should not read anything on the internet as he believed it would confuse her. Although she was not sure what road to take, she did not want to venture ignorantly into the system of surgery, chemotherapy and radiation treatments without proper consideration. She knew an informed decision was vital, as her life depended on it.

Acquiring knowledge on diet and a positive lifestyle is important. Well-defined, coherent information will give you the knowledge and know-how to influence your life for the better. Lack of education in this field can lead you to make wrong decisions. The need for more education on these subjects is vital, I often think of the millions that are spent on the general education of our children, and yet very little of that time and money is put into educating them on the one thing they must do for the rest of their lives – eat.

Our use of the internet – a new, democratic medium – reflects our desire for more information. The success of the 'University of Google' bears testament to our need for knowledge to feed our hungry minds. With this new information tool at our disposal, the possibility for better education on these subjects is now available to ordinary people like you and me. Those of us who search for health would do well to pay attention to the wealth of research showing that good nutrition is the best ally against diseases, including heart disease, cancer, diabetes and Crohn's disease.

Science and medicine plays a vital role in assisting our populations. The improvements in infant mortality and the incredible work carried out in A&E are prime examples of this, however we cannot ignore the root cause of problems in the treatment of diseases. It is not enough to treat symptoms, we must look into our diet and lifestyles to find causes. We should try to understand that this missing factor can lead us away from the problem or it can lead us right to the heart of it. All research, even at the microbiological level, demonstrates the benefit of maintaining health rather than waiting until we have a problem that needs to be fixed.

Aware that Amy and her doctor did not have a like-minded approach, I could see no way of opening the dialogue between them. Getting to the heart of the problem was not going to be easy without teamwork and collaboration especially as she was determined to find the source of the problem, and was no longer prepared to just treat the symptoms.

Of course, I do not interfere with patient's decisions to undergo conventional treatments, that is not my role. For some people there are major psychological benefits to having surgery, and chemotherapy and radiation treatments, as they feel that they have 'removed' the disease in a short time and this helps restore their all-important positive mental attitude. Many people choose to have conventional treatment after chatting with me but if addressing the underlying cause is their focus, I help them find ways to improve their diets and lifestyles.

Finally, Amy decided she would arm herself with the correct information.

As she did her best to understand and learn more about her illness by reading and by researching on the internet, she came across thousands of studies supporting the role of nutrition in healing disease, but she also found research in various publications that alleged there were beneficial monetary gains between pharmaceutical companies and the medical establishment. She immersed herself in the literature and amassed a great deal of information on these issues. Amy was so incensed with her findings that she was absolutely determined to 'tell it as it is'.

As she spoke of the confusing and frustrating ordeal she was going through, she asked, 'It's not unusual to tackle other illnesses such as heart disease with diet, so why are they so cynical about the connection between cancer and diet?'

Unwavering in her resolve to make sense of her findings, she questioned, 'Do they really want to find the solution to this disease when there is so much in it for them?'

As I spend my time empowering individuals to take control in their lives, it puts me at the frontline of these issues. Increasingly, I am finding these questions difficult to answer. I myself have benefited greatly from the dedication of my doctors and oncologist, however, I can see that much of their education is aimed towards drug solutions, not the workings of nature.

As these people deal directly with some of the most important decisions of our lives, they must realise that it is very disconcerting for a patient who has been diagnosed with cancer to know who to trust when they do their own research. I can't help thinking that a little more sensitivity and patience would have gone a long way towards helping Amy understand fully the risks and benefits of her treatment options. Perhaps if Amy's doctor had stood for a moment in her shoes, he may have seen things in a different light.

There are better approaches: a combination of understanding and co-operation between patient and doctor helps the patient make informed choices about their medical care. Ultimately, a new level of openness and transparency must be presented freely if we are to make a fundamental difference for patients who is evaluating his or her options.

Maybe the time has come to revamp the standard medical model, where compliance is expected. If we had a structured educational programme which encourages participation, interaction and collaboration, we could share knowledge effectively, counteract a lot of misinformation and help patients take responsibility for their health. A move like this could save the health service in the long run.

Prevention is Better than a Cure

My biggest problem with conventional medicine comes when prevention is ignored. Lifestyle, dietary and environmental factors need to be taken seriously. The National Cancer Institute statistics show that there were 12.9 million new cases diagnosed worldwide in 2009, theses are really scary statistics. When we consider this rise, we may well regret ignoring the potential of prevention. The institute's current director, John Niederhuber, noted that 'cancer is a global health crisis'.

A study by the International Agency for Research on Cancer states that:

> *In the developing world, cancers of the liver, stomach and esophagus are more common, they are often linked to consumption of carcinogenic, preserved foods, such as smoked or salted food, and parasitic infections that attack organs. Developed countries tended to have cancers linked to affluence or a 'Western lifestyle' – cancers of the colon, rectum, breast and prostate – that can be caused by obesity, lack of exercise, diet and age.*

Cancer rates appear to have increased dramatically since the Industrial Revolution. Before that, there are few indications of cancer in humans. If cancer rates today are at an all-time high, it stands to reason that we are doing something fundamentally wrong. If substantial progress is to be forthcoming, we need to look sufficiently at the role of prevention and shift the emphasis to lifestyle choices.

I am convinced that if we focus on strengthening the body's immune system to fight disease, there is a chance that all of us could reduce our risk of contracting these serious illnesses. Eating nutritious food could well be the most important health measure that any of us can take. Anyone who fears cancer can't afford to ignore this important fact if we are to create health for ourselves and our children. Those who have recovered from terminal illness know only too well how the body's healing systems improved their chances of recovery. I know many people who have stepped away from drug-orientated medical practices and have begun to think differently about the conventional way of dealing with disease.

Amy was prepared to take on this fight against her doctors and convention single-handedly. As an objective onlooker, I felt it was not sensible for her to allow herself to be side-tracked from her own healing by these issues – even though I always encourage my students to become informed as it helps them when evaluating their options; knowledge is power.

It's OK to be afraid, but fear should never stop you from getting answers. I believe strongly that you are at a serious disadvantage when you don't understand your disease – when you learn about your disease, you gain a better understanding of how to deal with it. Building an understanding of the origin and development of disease fosters awareness and responsibility for the person affected. It is also important to stay focused on your healing, the primary goal is to get well, not to change the world.

In this instance, the scale of Amy's health challenge had become obscured by her tenacious hunt to repudiate modern medicine's gains. While it was admirable that she wanted to right the wrongs, I felt that pursuing these issues would be to her detriment. Her first concern had to be her own survival. I knew she must develop a single-minded focus on her healing if she was to succeed.

Throughout her flurry of rebellion, I tried to defuse the situation and to rein in her urge to fight for her new beliefs. I gave her a push in the direction of the major challenge she was facing with her own health by advising her to focus on winning her battle with cancer, and to leave the war with the pharmaceutical companies to those who were in a position to effect change. Just as you cannot fight the forces of nature, I felt she was fighting a losing battle. It's always wise to choose your battles.

However deserving of praise Amy's intentions were, investigations and recriminations of this nature usually run into problems for the person involved. The reason being that one individual cannot effect change. The tragedy of Amy's story is her inability to find a middle ground when looking for a solution to this cruel and frightening disease we call cancer.

Throughout her deep, personal search for truth, Amy found out that there are a growing number of doctors who take a nutritional approach to treating disease. Those who have looked beyond conventional medicine in their search for health can feel vindicated by the work of the researchers and doctors who have dedicated their lives to achieving radical solutions to the treatment of serious illnesses.

Dr Philip Binzel is among those who have advocated nutrition in a medical setting. He was a pioneer and teacher and, although now officially retired, he practised medicine for over 40 years. While this provocative thinker had a successful career, he felt limited by the traditional confines of his profession. Binzel was a doctor who worked inside the system, when he tried to pursue truth as he knew it, his work with nutrition led him to take on the entire medical establishment.

When Binzel began to investigate nutrition, one of the main obstacles he encountered was a lack of nutritional knowledge. In his years of medical training, he had not received a single lecture on nutrition. Binzel had a willingness to learn and made it his priority to find out more about nutrition and prevention.

Binzel wrote in his book *Alive and Well* how he discovered the importance of enzymes and nitrilosides (vitamin B17) in the diet. He also found out that numerous nutritional deficiencies exist within the cancer patients. Binzel put together a nutritional programme for his patients that was easy to follow and he had exceptionally impressive results with the patients who adopted the dietary regime he prescribed. Many of Binzel's patients had previously been told by their doctors that they had no hope of surviving as their cancers were terminal. A high percentage of these patients remained *alive and well* many years later.

Another visionary in this field is health researcher Dr T. Colin Campbell. He also decided to step out of the system and disclose the truth about food. Dr Campbell explained to the American public:

> *As a taxpayer who foots the bill for research and health policy in America, you deserve to know that many of the common notions you have been told about food, health and disease are wrong.*

Campbell's research may be controversial, but his scientific reputation is indisputable.

Patrick Holford wrote in his book *Optimum Nutrition for the Mind*:

> *We must think our way out of the box, this means a new basis for both diagnosing and treating problems and a new way of eating that supports our health, rather than eroding it.*

Throughout my own research, I have come across many of these highly respected doctors who were part of a dedicated group voicing their beliefs, despite having to step outside the confines of their professions, such as Dr Ernesto Contreras, founder of the Oasis of Hope Hospital, and Professor Dean Burk, former head of the National Cancer Institute. These experts have worked for decades in specific areas to uncover major health truths that are not brought to the public's attention. They brought these issues out of the lab and the libraries and into real life where it belongs. Perhaps the thing that impressed me most in the large volume of material I had assimilated from these doctors was that they not only managed to think outside the box of established medicine, but they successfully made the information on key health issues available to the public at large.

To the Rescue

In the interim, Amy's oncology nurse stepped in – a very personable woman who was incredibly supportive and had a positive impact on her recovery. For Amy, she was the breath of fresh air she needed as she travelled down the conventional path. Apart from holding her hand and offering kind words of encouragement, this nurse realised that living in this confused state of mind would not aid Amy's recovery. She understood her fear of the unknown and her quest for answers in trying to make sense of everything she was hearing and reading. Having encountered these feelings with many other patients, the nurse set about assisting Amy to deal with the multitude of questions running through her mind.

This provided Amy with a support system that reassured her throughout her treatment. She presented a very different face to her nurse, and was able to speak with her in a way that she never would have to her doctor. It was a lifeline that set her mind to rest, and she settled into her treatment plan, while also working to change her lifestyle and eating habits.

Amy is alive and well on the road to recovery, and wrote to me recently that:

I am feeling healthy, energetic, and better than I have felt in years. I am really indebted to my oncology nurse, her awareness of my concerns and emotional standing helped me get my head together. Her knowledge and understanding that the whole-food approach was a natural way to heal my body inspired confidence in me. It was refreshing to find someone whose views closely matched my own. I wouldn't be where I am today without her help. Many of the naturopathy and homeopathy therapies I opted for resonated with her at a core level. These alternative therapies really helped me through my treatment. Don't let anyone tell you that they have no value. My doctor is impressed by my rapid recovery, he is pleased with my scan results, but shows no interest in my new regime.

Chapter Twelve

Investing in the Future

∽

'Dream big dreams, but never forget that realistic short-term goals are the keys to your success.'

MAC ANDERSON

Over the past decade, many countries have experienced unprecedented economic growth. For a time, house building reached record levels and, certainly within the more affluent areas, there was a surge in the number of people purchasing country homes, apartments, holiday homes abroad and investment properties.

Now, imagine for a moment the money, time and commitment, not to mention the energy, it takes to set up an additional property. If we were to invest and funnel that same level of resources into our health, isn't it likely that we could expect to offset the burden of the inevitable downward spiral of ill-health we experience as we age? Certainly, we live longer today, but the truth is that the latter half of our lives is often stacked up with a host of health problems. These are the facts, not scare tactics.

In spite of these problems, we continue to hide from the truth and we make ruthless cutbacks in the time we invest in our health. It is commonplace to subsidise our diets with junk food and all manner of convenience foods. These foods are certainly handy and easy to prepare, but these shortcuts do not provide foods that will nourish the human body. The adverse effects associated with lifestyles built around this food trap are well known and publicised. Yet, we convince ourselves that these neglectful lifestyles will have no consequences to our overall health. We come up with every imaginable reason why these energy-zapping foods are a necessity, but this denial is nothing short of shooting ourselves in the foot.

Clearly, not all of us are guilty of this, but this recipe for confusion successfully manages to condemn us to a large range of health problems. Well, maybe the time has come when we need to wake up and not continue down this road of self-sabotage, the result of which is exorbitant fees paid out for treatments and medical care when things go wrong. It's enough to send you into financial ruin.

Sickness is at the heart of a very profitable multibillion dollar industry. For the over-burdened taxpayer who pours money into our deteriorating healthcare system, the absence of an emphasis on preventative healthcare can weigh heavily. The high demand for and increasing constraints on these health services could be substantially reduced if we employed some preventative measures.

You may not be sick enough to take to your bed with, for example, insomnia, digestive problems or respiratory complaints but, surely, it is foolish to rely on others to bail us out when we have the ability to nip these health problems in the bud. In light of the deepening crisis within our health services, it makes perfect sense to hold on to your most valuable asset – your health. After all, is it wise to become dependent on a health service that is finding it difficult to deliver a comprehensive service to its patients? Crisis management does not instil confidence.

If you are serious about your health, then there is a better way. Prevention is always better than a cure – it's cheap, effective and, best of all, there is no risk involved. It has a high impact on your health and you can have the best of both worlds. You will have the rewards of increased energy levels and better health, plus you will no longer be dependent on our weakening health services. It's a low-cost, effective way of recharging your batteries and produces a guaranteed return on the time invested.

The Japanese are fully aware of the knock-on effect of self-care measures and employ numerous health-promoting incentives within their workforce. During the Cultural Revolution in China, when doctors were taken from their posts, the people were forced to practise chi gung every day. It was the law. Those in power recognised that self-care was important for the people.

Get interested in your health before you have to. Prevention begins with you. Make your biggest investment in the one place you must live for the rest of your life – your body. Don't wait for a wake-up call.

Martin's Wake-Up Call

Martin is a successful businessman who has a considerable repertoire of talents. He is self-employed, multi-skilled and holds numerous qualifications. In the early years of building his business, Martin was his own administrator, marketing guru, IT expert and bookkeeper all rolled into one. He spent his life trying to be one-step ahead of the game and had a strong drive to succeed and, by the age of 40, had built an impressive business.

Although his hectic lifestyle was now becoming financially rewarding, it was also exhausting. Despite his fatigue, he was driven to achieve. He was very much a part of today's chaotic rat race: a workaholic – running himself ragged, eating on the run, arriving home late most evenings, with weekends inevitably spent sorting out some crisis or other. Martin was working himself to the bone and functioning on adrenalin. People, who exist on adrenalin, don't know when to slow down. Not only are these lifestyles difficult to sustain, they are also addictive. Martin considered sleep a waste of productive time and prided himself on surviving on four hours of rest a night.

Even though he now had a team of good, loyal people behind him, life continued to produce a never-ending cycle of pressures and problems for Martin. He was stretched in all directions and, like many others in today's world, he had become a slave to his success. The looming deadlines and high-pressure conditions he worked under were a normal part of the job. The leisure activities that he used to enjoy, such as golf or lounging around watching football, were out of the question.

He explained that, in hindsight, if he was to be completely honest, he knew deep down that working in this environment for many years had short-changed his health. However, he felt trapped and did not know how he could escape. The bottom line was that he felt compelled to keep it all going. The pressure for financial success came with a heavy price tag.

Unfortunately for Martin, there were storm clouds on the horizon. Just as he was starting to see the fruits of his labour, life dealt him a severe blow. He had been seeing a haematologist for several years, receiving treatment for high platelets, for which he had been told there was no cause. There were no outward symptoms of his disorder, although the medication he was taking was causing some side effects. Nevertheless, he had learned to live with them and was getting on with his life.

He first learned his disease was fatal when his life insurance doubled in price. When he moved house in 2005, his haematologist disclosed some facts to the life-insurance company that he had neglected to tell Martin. When Martin queried why his life insurance costs had risen, he was advised to talk to his doctor. He contacted his doctor who promptly brushed the issue aside saying, 'You know insurance companies – they'll rip you off at every corner.'

He went back to the insurer and asked them to justify the rise in price and was, once again, referred back to his doctor. But he got the same response as before – and this continued for nine months until a, by-now exasperated, underwriter at the life-insurance company told Martin that they had received a fax from his doctor saying that things had changed with Martin's health. The underwriter explained he had no authority to divulge that type of information, but he knew how frustrated Martin must be feeling at being sent round in circles.

When Martin went back to the haematologist with this bit of information, the doctor denied at first that there was any such letter, but then he acknowledged that he had sent something to the insurer. Martin was rendered speechless when he was told that his disorder had become terminal 18 months earlier and that he had approximately five years to live.

His condition had escalated into myelofibrosis, a rare condition that affects the bone marrow and which only responds to a few drugs, including an agrilide drug (a platelet-reducing agent) that turned out to be the most successful at controlling his platelets. However, the haematologist explained that one of the side effects of this drug is that it accelerates the disorder, and, by this stage, Martin had been taking it for seven years. The other option Martin had was to take Hydrea, a chemotherapeutic drug, which has skin cancer and secondary leukaemia listed amongst its side effects. These drugs were the only ones offered to help control the symptoms of his disease until the 'inevitable bone marrow transplant, or death'.

His doctor rated Martin's chance of surviving the bone-marrow transplant at about 20 per cent. For Martin, it was like a bolt out of the blue. Telling his wife Aishling was agonising, as he felt that he was abandoning her in the world. He resolved to double his efforts at work so that she would have no financial worries after he was gone. Her response was that they should take charge of the situation and invest their efforts in finding a way to help him survive.

When Aishling asked the haematologist if there was anything they could do to help Martin, she was told that there wasn't. She had always been an advocate of healthy living and believed that food had nutritional and healing benefits, so she asked the haematologist his opinion about the benefits of good nutrition on Martin's condition. He said that Martin should probably eat a few green vegetables. She asked about stress, but the doctor dismissed it out of hand, saying that it had no impact on well-being. They left his office without getting direction or hope.

Although Martin was desperately trying to put on a brave face, the news shocked him to his core. A feeling of disbelief followed by a spiral of worries flooded in on top of him – a common response to such shocking news. Martin never thought this would happen to him. He mistakenly believed that as he was young, reasonably fit, had never struggled with his weight and had never smoked, surely it meant that the law of averages was on his side. There were the few pints of beer with the lads on a Friday night, but that was his only vice.

Of course, his friends and family had warned him he was working too hard and now all those years of successful denial caught up with him. Aishling could see the problem for what it really was; that a great gulf existed between the time he invested on his work and on his personal life. She viewed this wake-up call as a signal, a red flag that he desperately needed to change direction in his life. Now that he had come so close to the wire, it made her realise that everything had to change, he could no longer take his health for granted. This was a life and death struggle and he was going to have to confront it with all the weapons in his armoury. She agreed they really needed to remove the major stressors from his life.

Anxious to hasten his progress, Aishling persuaded Martin to see a naturopath where he was put on a detox diet which helped enormously with the side effects of the drugs. However, the disorder still progressed at a steady pace.

Changing his Priorities

They knew they had to 'up their game', but they did not know how. Some years earlier, Aishling had introduced herself to me and we connected instantly, from which a wonderful friendship took off. The common-sense steps of my programme resonated with her and she adopted many of them into her daily life with ease. Martin, on the other hand, had dismissed them. He couldn't see the sense in it and, anyway, he was far too busy. Now he had nowhere else to turn, but he couldn't get his head around 'how a couple of vegetables were going to fix what the well-educated doctors could not reverse'. Aishling arranged for him to meet with me to discuss the rationale of my programme as well as the regime. He told her he wanted some time to think about it.

Naturally, Aishling wanted to save him, but she knew that this was Martin's decision, one that only he could make. My experience has taught me that if the individual is not open to changing their ways, then it will not happen. Everything and anything will get in their way – they will be too busy or too tired to accomplish the simple tasks necessary for them to change their lives. It's easy to become trapped in a mindset that stands between success and achievement. Your mindset is the deciding factor in success or failure. Loved ones, family and friends may want a person to change to give them a better life, but if that person is not ready for it, all their efforts will produce poor results. Rarely can we control another person's behaviour.

Although I cautioned Martin that he needed to concentrate on getting better and should not allow work to interfere with his ability to respond to his treatment and recovery, I also recommended to Aishling that she give him a few days to take it all in. In the end, he might come round to her way of thinking. Even though the road he had to embark on was going to be rocky, in my heart I felt sure that Martin would see the way forward. This was his chance – possibly his one and only chance – to save his life.

As Martin prepared for the inevitable treatments that lay ahead, Aishling tried hard to persuade him to take a back seat in the business for a while. Eventually, he agreed. Of course, Martin knew this made perfect sense, but he openly admitted that even in the face of a threat to his existence, he could not imagine how he could step back and relinquish control of the business he had worked so hard to build.

However, a life-threatening illness has a way of influencing your priorities. The crisis of illness is often the primary agent of change. For some, the motivation factor has to be big in order to bring about lifestyle change. Love is one of the greatest motivators of all and it was evident to me how deeply Martin and Aishling cared for each other.

Aishling was enormously relieved and reassured by Martin's decision. She did not want him to rely entirely on the medical establishment as they had offered them no hope. In conjunction with his treatment, she wanted Martin to follow a combination of alternative and nutritional routes. As she saw it, he had a choice – to do as the haematologist told him and wait and see whether he lived or died, or to find out everything he could about how to save his life. There was no time to waste and he had to sit up and take notice. Her enthusiasm was infectious. Clearly, she understood that he could not afford to get it wrong.

Martin was adamant that Aishling should not fuss, but I could see through the silly, nervous banter between them that she could not bear the thought of losing him. They had a wonderfully supportive relationship. I found her a very perceptive woman, there was strength about her character, she was a leader, and leaders are not afraid to fail. I suspect he will never know how much of a life saver she really was to him.

On that first visit, when Martin was finding it hard to face the sudden threat of death; I did not want to bombard him with intrusive questions. He spoke very openly to me, explaining how, as an engineer, he was a very factual type of person and had very little room for grey areas, tending to see things in black or white. However, with so much conflicting information out there, he asked if I could cut to the chase and steer him in the right direction. He wanted the full facts on how my programme worked, the research behind it and how much time it would take to implement. He also asked me what guarantees I could offer if he was to make the effort required. I asked him to recall what the haematologist had promised him. He nodded and I could see his resolve harden.

Investment in Life

When confronted with a major health challenge, knowledge is vital. I totally understood Martin's need for more information and his sense of urgency. We chatted for a while and, in plain language, I explained that the basic principle of my programme is to kick start the immune system and boost the defence functions of the body. An overworked, depleted immune system is not capable of healing.

I made it clear that the more support you give to the immune system, the better your chance of fighting disease and handling any possible side effects of treatments. I explained that, just like a car, the body has certain requirements and needs the correct fuel in order to function properly.

A typical day for Martin was a mad dash into work with a piece of toast in his hand, bolting down a sandwich at lunch time if he had a minute, dinner at around nine in the evening, and, of course, coffee, coffee, coffee. We agreed it was not a recipe for health. I pointed out to Martin that malnourished people do not make good candidates for healing. I also pointed out that it was going to take more than a new dietary regime to turn this situation around. He also needed to get his head around this new lifestyle, as lifestyle choices also influence the immune system.

Over the years, I have become very aware that aligning our thoughts for change is an absolute necessity if we are to achieve a positive outcome. In a bid to get Martin to identify the habitual negative choices he had been making and start to eliminate them from his life, I explained he had to look at all aspects of his life as a full package. I made it clear that without this, he would be merely putting a band-aid over the problem.

Thankfully, this concept was not a bridge too far for Martin and he seemed to understand its relevance perfectly. I also did my best to encourage him to remember that his level of success would be dependant solely on how much time and effort he invested. As with any project, you get out what you put in. Shoring up his commitment would require Martin to be consistently active in feeding the needs of his body. I believe strongly that actions speak louder than words. A proactive and positive attitude would put him back in the driving seat. Research shows that negative or positive actions send messages to the immune system. His body would depend on him to deliver.

Aishling and I had high hopes that Martin would invest the same effort into his health as he had his business. I am relieved to say that this is what happened. Eventually, Martin declared his resolve to try to regain his health and from that moment on, he did not flinch from carrying his decision through. It was a crucial decision that was to totally transform his life.

Although he was a first-timer, he took on the steps of The Programme without any problems. Aishling already had converted their shopping trolley into an organic-only zone and had installed a water filtration system some years earlier. She now added sprouting to their regime and Martin took over the juicing and, surprisingly, developed a taste for a vegetarian diet. He fitted it in alongside his treatment and found it supported the problems he encountered with the treatment wonderfully.

As he embraced each additional element of the programme, he said that he felt like each step was stacking the odds in his favour. Aishling introduced one step at a time, until it became ingrained into his daily routine. When he was tempted by junk food or had cravings for treats, she found healthy substitutes to exchange for their regular food choices. She became somewhat of an expert in focusing on the foods they could eat (as opposed to what they couldn't). This simple tactic changed the way they ate because they did not feel deprived of the food they normally ate.

The drugs were very hard on his digestive tract and Martin suffered many side effects, one of which was chronic diarrhoea. During the treatment, he used green juices and enzymes to help him break up the food he ate and this eased the problem. He found a strong probiotic that replaced good bacteria in the mouth to help him recover from the sore mouth ulcers he was experiencing. The disease progressed aggressively for a further five months and he had a few more problems on the way, hitting a huge low as he struggled to get through the day. As he had told nobody except family and a few very close friends about his illness, he had to attempt to make things look 'normal'. This wasn't easy as the disease took its toll on his weight and energy.

Team Effort

However, Martin had a will of iron and Aishling was there every step of the way, researching the programme, especially the parts that they didn't understand at first, and presented the main facts to him as clearly as she could. Her understanding and complete involvement in what he was going through, meant that they could discuss all the elements of his healing. There is so much information available that it was important to have somebody to tease it out with.

They were relieved when Aishling learned that his apparent dis-improvement may well have been what is called a 'healing crisis' and is very often part of the body's natural recovery. When she researched further, she found that the weight loss could be down to the body's way of dumping toxic cells and his lack of energy was possibly the body diverting its resources into healing and thereby a way of forcing him to relax.

They looked into many complementary therapies and Martin worked with a traditional Chinese doctor and a bio-energy therapist at various stages to help him deal with the side effects of the drugs and with the symptoms of his healing crises. Martin still refers to his Chinese doctor as Dr Voodoo, but it's very much tongue in cheek as he knows how beneficial this doctor has been to his recovery. The bio-energist worked wonders with his circulation as she rebalanced his energy and restored warmth to his icy cold hands and feet. Once they had become open to nutritional healing, it raised the bar and opened them up to a world of options that had seemed a little crazy at first, but transpired to be of great benefit without the invasive effects of chemicals.

Whenever things appeared to be going badly, such as when Martin's platelets soared sky high or a hernia problem developed, he and his wife would talk over the alternatives that conventional medicine had to offer. However, they decided that relying on strong drugs with horrible side effects was not an option for them. They were both determined to get away from anything that was suppressing his immune system. Their unifying purpose channelled all their energies into getting Martin better. It was a real team effort and we all know that teams make fewer mistakes.

Approximately five months into the new regime, they noticed that the deep wrinkles that Martin had had for many years had softened dramatically and that the grey hair at his temples had reverted to brown once more. While these were welcome changes, they were not excited for reasons of vanity. They knew from their research that the body doesn't heal selectively, and if the outward visible elements were renewing, then the same changes must be taking place inside.

As he deepened his commitment to the process and lost his scepticism, things improved quite a bit, resulting in Martin celebrating his new-found energy by overdoing it at the gym and tearing a muscle. Thankfully, his general well-being had taken a leap forward and his muscle healed quickly. Soon afterwards, he was back at the gym and he also bought a bicycle to commute to work.

After just 10 months on The Programme, Martin's platelets returned to normal. They had not been at that level since 2002. The haematologist could not believe it – he said Martin should be in an acute leukaemic state.

The part of this mind-body approach that Martin struggled with most was the relaxation element. He has dabbled with yoga, tai chi and meditation in an attempt to still his busy mind and has certainly made some progress in this area, but this is an aspect of his healing that he is still working on.

Over the following year, Martin and Aishling stayed in touch with me, and the following is an extract from an email Aishling sent to me recently:

> *Martin is on top of the world and really well. Sticking to The Programme has become so much easier now that we've started seeing results. I feel foolish now in saying that it appeared to be a mammoth task to get on top of. But your knowledge and understanding of the entire process is an amazing resource. Having the healing crises explained to us was such a relief when we were afraid of the deep sores, the hernia and the rashes that erupted. It helped us stay calm knowing that mood swings and long weak spells, where Martin was unable to climb the stairs without pain, were part of the clearing and rejuvenation process. Your gentle no-nonsense approach has helped us stay strong and committed. You never allowed us to make excuses for ourselves, or to let ourselves off lightly. The life of hope you introduced us to replaced the cloud of fear we lived under. There is no downside to having hope. It gives us a reason to strive.*

On follow-up conversations with Martin, he acknowledged that the active role he took in his treatment influenced his recovery and tipped the scales in his favour. He felt that taking the time to invest in his health was the single most important step of his life. Because Martin came so close to the edge, he found the focus to do what was necessary. He has not reverted back to old habits. He makes time each day for physical exercise, prepares his juice before he leaves for work and when he gets home in the evening.

He is a very sociable guy and was concerned that he would not fit in with the lads in the pub. Drinking water rather than a few pints was an embarrassment for him initially. The last thing he wanted was to stand out from the crowd. But these issues seemed irrelevant when he became conversant with the drawbacks to his health of his 'one vice'. His friends soon became accepting of his preference to avoid alcohol and no longer comment on it.

Martin still travels quite a lot, and eating out presented another problem. When he pulled into a filling station and came face to face with an attractive display of chocolate, he soon found he was drawn back into his old ways. When he gave in to temptation, he would spend his time beating himself up for giving in. What has really helped him stay on track has been making friends with a few like-minded, positive people. Socialising with these people has been a great help to him because healthy eating is normal for them. With his regular gym sessions, he is slowly rebuilding muscle weight and no longer looks gaunt. He is back playing golf and takes some well deserved weekend breaks with Aishling.

He is now a guy who totally 'walks his talk' when it come to healthy living. His proactive approach vastly improved the quality of not just his health (no small feat) but also his life. This life-threatening illness was the catalyst that helped restore balance to Martin's busy life.

Chapter Thirteen

Old Habits Die Hard

*'To keep the body in good health is a duty ... otherwise we shall
not be able to keep our mind strong and clear.'*

BUDDHA

Food glorious food, is it our friend or our enemy? Eating good
food is an immensely pleasurable experience and as food is
the cornerstone of my programme, this chapter is about removing
habits and beliefs that interfere with your ability to get to grips
with changing your lifestyle.

Our food habits are programmed into us from an early age; as a
result, we develop good and bad habits surrounding food. The
food we eat has an important impact on how we feel, yet many of
us have a love–hate relationship with food that dominates a large
part of our eating habits.

Eating habits have the power to create health or destroy it. As my
mother would say as she stuffed cabbage into me as a child, 'If
you don't eat well, you won't live well.' Foods are the body's major
source of nutrients and we must obtain these essential nutrients

from our foods if we want to optimise health and reverse many of the symptoms of disease. If we don't, our bodies will gradually fall apart. When we eat good food, we support the body's basic needs and functions.

In most instances, we get sick from lifestyle-related issues. As you have read in previous chapters, our lifestyle choices can have a direct influence on our immune systems. Naturally, we pay little attention to our health when it is good, but when illness arises, it soon becomes very clear that we need to change the direction of our lifestyle, including the foods we eat. If we become complacent and cut corners with our health, how long will it be before the body decides it's payback time?

I know it's not always easy to get the balance right, especially if you work long hours and are trying to juggle work and family commitments. Sometimes, you have barely the time to draw breath, let alone prepare a meal. If you are working and looking after a family, reaching for a less than healthy option often becomes the reality. Preparing the healthy option usually gets shoved down the list of priorities. There is nothing like the pressures of work and family to make you break all the rules of healthy living.

The questions to be asked are whether or not these shortcuts are proving to be a menace to our health. What will the consequences of these short-sighted decisions be? At what point must we put healthy eating practices in place? These questions are not just good discussion points, they are areas that need to be addressed if we are to achieve good health.

Many of us cling to social conditioning which says that a little of what you fancy does you good. This attitude is like a brick wall standing in our way. When we start to question our thinking about food, we realise this mental block is there because we put it there. Thoughts, beliefs, feelings and mental attitudes are important factors when it comes to food. Once we become aware of them, we begin to understand the power they have over our eating patterns.

Redefining what we Think

We need to change our thinking about the foods we eat.

I got a taste of this when I tried to give up sugar. It's a well known fact that sugar feeds fungus, yeasts, bacteria and even cancer. Yes, cancer cells thrive on sugar; cancer cells have many more receptor cells for capturing sugar than healthy cells. The molecular biology of cancer cells requires more glucose to feed them, and they meet their energy needs by fermentation. This is evident with the new and expensive medical procedure called PET (Positron Emission Tomography).

The PET scan is designed to detect any mass that is growing fast and it has the ability to identify tumours in their early phase. It works when a glucose molecule, which has been tagged with a small amount of radioactive element known as FDG (fluoro-deoxyglucose, the principal radiotracer for clinical PET imaging), is injected into the body. The glucose and radiotracer is absorbed by the cancer cells and the cancer cells can be identified and their activity monitored by this type of nuclear medicine imaging. Cutting down on our intake of sugar cuts off an important food supply to the cancer cells. For some people, cancer cells grow faster and stronger when the person's sugar levels are frequently above normal.

Yet sugar and chocolate are synonymous with pleasure; such is its sweet temptation that we ignore the devastating effects it has on our health. This is a big mistake. Today's Western diet is laced with sugary foods. Large amounts of sugars are found in cakes, muffins, biscuits, chocolate and other sweets. These are just a few of the sugar-laced foods that we have acquired a taste for, but such refined carbohydrates are like a time bomb ticking within our systems. Even white bread and pasta that are staple foods today are digested so fast that they act like sugar within the system.

So how can we deal with such an addiction? Have you ever actually tried to give it up? Be warned; it's not easy. Sugar is one of the most addictive substances to break free from. When I discovered exactly how bad this sweet poison really was for my health, I had no choice but to trade in my sweet tooth for a more discerning mouthful. So I began to play around with the idea of attaching some negative thoughts to my little treats. Every time I fancied a piece of chocolate or a sticky bun, I told myself that this was feeding cancer, destroying my teeth, putting on extra weight and causing major imbalances in my body. This may seem a bit over the top, but if sugar is strong enough to penetrate through tooth enamel, can you imagine the damage it can cause within your body?

Adding a negative association to food can change the way you think about it. It is well recognised as a useful mental tool to help those wanting to kick harmful habits. Developing feelings of revulsion towards the foods you are compelled towards can be a simple yet very powerful way of giving up those foods – for example, imagine your favourite chocolate bar tastes like a food you hate. When you see your sugar habit from this perspective, it soon begins to lose its attraction.

Even so, these habits are not always controlled by rational thinking. Despite the consequences for my health, I still felt desperately hard done by going without my fix. While I knew that every time I ate these refined sugary foods they caused an imbalance in body chemistry and my unfortunate body was faced with the challenge of trying to restore a state of equilibrium. I tried to delude myself that I needed just a little something sweet to keep my blood sugars stable.

Of course this was nonsense, because far from maintaining sugar levels all it did was push my system into overload by keeping my blood sugars on a constant roller coaster of highs and lows. The type of energy we obtain from sugary junk food is short-lived and causes a fast rise in blood sugar levels that is usually followed by an abrupt slump. You enter a relentless cycle. This constant yo-yoing between high and low blood sugar levels gives us short-lived energy. The result is that we end up worn out, burned out and exhausted. It's not just your long-suffering teeth that are affected – refined sugars have been connected to a host of diseases, including diabetes, cancer, arthritis, heart disease, Crohn's disease and obesity.

Not only is the energy derived from sugar short-lived, the satisfaction it gives us is too. As a result, we go back again and again for more and more. I knew that these foods were bound to leave their mark on my health and while I did not want to admit this at first. I realised that if I could not alter my diet, then I would only perpetuate a situation I wanted to change. As Albert Einstein said 'insanity is doing the same thing over and over again and expecting different results'.

Despite the mouth-watering pleasures, I decided I was not going to surrender to the melt-in-the-mouth products any more. Knowing only too well that the spirit can be willing, but the flesh is weak, I realised that if I was to make a consistent change it had to come from within.

Easier said than done, you might say, and at the time these were my sentiments too. I was definitely not looking forward to breaking free of my little pleasures. OK I could do it for a week or two, but eventually I would slip back into having 'just a little treat' and then I would be hooked once more. The prospect of the sugar blues seemed daunting, but if I changed my thinking about my little treats by attaching negative thoughts to sugar, maybe I would stand a chance of overcoming the cravings.

Cultivating Good Habits

It takes some time to create these habits – so naturally it was going to take time to undo them. But cultivating good habits can help you improve your chances of long-term success. Initially, I fought off the urge for sugar by allowing myself a weekend treat, just to get myself over the hump. I had often used this tactic with the kids when they were young, so I decided I would reverse the psychology and see if I could manage to do the same.

It helps train the mind to adjust and you become less dependent on your sugar treats. The secret is to make it a treat not a habit and to find healthy substitutes. I learned to make treats from almonds, raisins and coconut. For a while I still craved something sweet, but I am now able to resist the temptation. I even managed to win my husband over; he was a self-confessed chocoholic and had a very sweet tooth.

In order to overcome the momentary pleasures of sugar, I have always found it a good idea to find alternatives and add them to my diet before eliminating the foods that I am already used to.

Another tip to prevent sugar cravings is to try natural plant sweeteners, like stevia and cinnamon, to replace refined sugars. Stevia is about 4 times sweeter than sugar and is credited with potentially positive health effects. A plant native to South America it is now grown and cultivated throughout the world as a replacement for sugars. Chlorella supplements are also useful in helping you to get over your craving as it helps balance blood sugars. Blood sugar regulation of (hyper/hypo) glycemic episodes is essential if you are to succeed in getting rid of your sweet tooth.

I must admit that it takes time to phase out sugary treats, but, eventually, you will lose your sweet tooth. As the desire passes, you will find sugar no longer has the same attraction it once had.

By finding a few tricks to help me tackle my sugar addiction, I managed to move my comfort zone. I found the most straight-forward way to stop eating these sugary foods was to change my thinking. As my mind supported my intention not to eat these foods, the desire to eat them began to fade. As the work progressed in helping my husband lose his sweet tooth, he took the initiative and visited a hypnotherapist. There was no chance that he would expend a lot of time or energy trying to give up his addiction to chocolate, he wanted a quick fix.

Hypnotic induction works on a subconscious level and has many advantages for those wanting to control panic attacks, anxiety, to quit smoking or lose weight, and manage phobias, eating problems, drinking and insomnia. Overcoming the mental blocks that are often triggered by internal factors such as stress can help control these problems.

Hypnosis is a wakeful state of focused attention that takes a bit of mental concentration, but this is easy with the guidance of a therapist who will help you stay focused so your mind does not wander off. Ger described it as a deep state of relaxation, although he had his doubts that he was in a trance state as his mind did wander about. The therapist will help you eliminate distractions and will customise the suggestions to your preferences in order to create a specific outcome. The heightened suggestibility of this therapy supercharges your state of consciousness to unleash the power of your mind to make a change for the better. The therapist can help you remove unwanted habits that relate to unhealthy foods and create a strong desire for wholesome foods. Hypnotherapy can also boost your mood and healing.

This hypnotic experience certainly changed Ger's chocolate addiction, and now, two and a half years on, he rarely craves chocolate. This is no mean feat for a man who had eaten six or seven bars of chocolate every day of his life. The results of this method of changing thought patterns speak for themselves. The added bonus is he no longer has weight issues.

Speaking of weight, this seems like and apt time to discuss diets.

Diets and Dieting

Up to one third of men and women in the Western world battle with their weight and with dieting, if we were to believe the media that figure would be closer to the entire population. The hard evidence suggests that food has become our enemy. Why is it the enemy when eating good food is such a wonderfully pleasurable experience? It is because we in the developed world have managed to turn this pleasure into junk binge eating.

If we continue to overfeed ourselves and ignore the impact of our unhealthy, Western diet, we will subject ourselves to the misery of the increasing epidemic of food-related diseases. When I asked my readers their opinion on this issue, there appeared to be two types of response. The main response centred on dieting; the other was based on health.

Readers' Responses to Diets

Even though people felt diets were a nightmare, they were drawn towards them like a magnet. This is possibly due to the unrelenting media attention on modern dietary habits; it's a huge focal point these days. They admitted they were easily seduced by the latest diet to come along and at the drop of a hat they switched from one diet to the next, hoping that this would be the one that would help them shed those extra pounds.

Who could blame them, especially when they are led to believe they can drop a dress size in two weeks or, better still, achieve that all-important flat stomach. With offers like this on the table, of course people will jump in feet first, hoping that they will reap the benefits of attaining the body they have always dreamed of.

But why do we bother to pursue the various diets that we are bombarded with when there is overwhelming evidence that diets do not work? If the diets we invest so much time and energy in are not always what they are cracked up to be, why do we continue to succumb to the outlandish claims of the advertisers?

We have become slaves to diets such as the Atkins Diet, the Scarsdale Diet and the South Beach Diet. These diets attract huge attention and make good stories for the media. The facts remain clear that eating less has become big business. We spent vast amounts of time and money trying to fathom the simple rules of weight loss. Is it any wonder that an entire industry has been built around it? It is truly a black mark against us that we have become incapable of recognising the hard sell.

Maybe we need to be a bit more discerning of the latest fad that catches our attention and become less willing to fall for the advertising and hype. Evaluating the ideal diet has become dauntingly complex, it's like negotiating your way through a minefield, and the confusion usually leads back to addictive comfort foods. Apart from the fact that all this binging and dieting is not healthy for your spirits, the disappointment we experience when we fail to see results we were expecting from a diet is deflating to say the least. You may know this to be true from first-hand experience.

The good news is that dieting becomes a thing of the past when you move to a healthier way of eating. This I discovered quite by accident when I changed my lifestyle. When I made the switch to nutritious foods, I visibly lost fat from underneath my chin, from my upper arms and all round my middle. I didn't actually drop much in weight; it was just that it became better spread on my body. This was a great change from all the other times that I tried various fad diets where I somehow managed to lose weight from all the places I didn't want to.

I am now in my fifties and at long last can forget the struggle of being able to fit into the jeans I always wanted to wear. For as long as I can remember, I have spent my life trying to squeeze, shove and pull my way into jeans. I now have the figure I wanted for most of my life and there has been no dieting, no guilt and most definitely no starvation diets. It was not that I was greatly overweight, but I had a few extra pounds here and there that I was always trying to lose. For 11 years I have managed to maintain a healthy weight and, thankfully, I have lost my middle-aged spread.

One of the best strategies you can employ if you feel you are overweight is to train your eating habits and to put more nourishing foods onto the menu. The latest low-carb craze makes you feel miserable because it robs you of the foods you need to give you energy. We need small amounts of carbohydrates, that should be eaten early in the day so they can be used to supply energy to do the things we need to do in the course of the day, but if carbohydrates are eaten late and don't get burned up for energy, they will be stored as fat. These types of fad diet only serve to make you feel deprived and hard done by when you deny yourself the foods you really want to eat.

The nutritional confusion about these diets is bad news for those who decide to follow them. As small amounts of fats and carbohydrates are an intrinsic part of a healthy body, it is not only our figures that suffer from abstaining from these foods but also our health. What goes into your mouth has a direct bearing on your health and your figure, so choose wisely. A balanced diet is the only way to go.

Readers' Responses on Health

Losing weight took precedence over health with a high percentage of those who responded, many of them admitted they had taken weight-loss pills. Food is more powerful than weight-loss pills will ever be and it has the ability to make us thin or fat, healthy or sick, depending on which foods we eat – don't underestimate its power.

Health may not have been an overriding factor when it came to food but as research shows there are consequences to the food we put into our mouths each day. In one particular study carried out by Dr Colin Campbell (*The China Study*), the results were startling, as he explained: 'It was a 100 to 0 score, leaving no doubt that nutrition trumped chemical carcinogens, even very potent carcinogens, in controlling cancer.'

If we continue with our bad habits and ignore the evidence, then, inevitably, it will limit our options to eat more healthily. We are habitually conditioned to using foods that are stripped of nutrients and this leaves us with an exhausted immune system. As the immune cells determine our state of health, the result of continually using these foods is that we become increasingly susceptible to disease, because the body loses its ability to repair itself.

Eating depleted food does not go unnoticed by the body and nature finds a way of fighting back. As a consequence of our poor food choices, the process of accelerated ageing occurs because the body cannot rejuvenate or regenerate cells as it needs to. Many of the illnesses and complaints we have come to accept today could be avoided by incorporating into our diets the foods our bodies require.

The term 'healthy food' may strike terror into your taste buds or conjure up an image of a leaf of lettuce and a stick of carrot for dinner. But don't panic, this negative connotation towards healthy food will soon disappear when you begin to taste how delicious this food can actually be.

The Mental Battle

Another area I became intrigued with was the interrelationship of emotions with the foods we eat. Obviously when we look at weight management, we can definitely establish a link with food and emotions but what is less often considered is the vital role that emotions play in health matters. We all want to be healthy but habits and emotions can often stand in our way. It's logical that when we struggle emotionally, it becomes a lot easier to reach for the 'quick fix'. If you frequently find yourself reaching for something to eat to relieve unwanted emotional states, you must ask yourself if you are using food rationally to nourish your body or if it has become an emotional crutch.

Being bored, sad, lonely or anxious can often trigger food cravings. One reader explained: 'If I am bored or anxious I eat everything in sight, especially if I have been eating well for a few days, I tell myself I deserve it because I have been so good. It's a constant mental battle.'

If this has hit a nerve or is ringing any alarm bells for you, it may be time to tackle your modus operandi, your health is too precious to use in such a way.

One indicator of this problem's reach might be the explosive growth in obesity we have seen over the past few decades. We are rapidly moving in the same direction as America. Food can numb painful feelings, ease mood swings, stop us feeling lonely or simply help us pass the time when we are bored. Perhaps we are reluctant to confront the internal conflict we have about the foods we eat. Even so, my suggestion for dealing with these mental battles is to call a truce – I did and it worked. Find nourishing foods that will appeal to your taste buds. There are tons of simple recipes out there, including my own, that will help you make delicious tasty dishes for you and your family. Once you fix in your mind that you will do it and succeed, the process becomes easier, but that mental decision is a must and there is no way around it.

Bear in mind that it is difficult to change the eating habits of a lifetime, particularly if you are not motivated by some particular reason. For some, changing their eating habits will always be a bridge too far; for others, it is a lifeline that moves them on to a better life. Instead of being discouraged by changing your eating habits, why not build upon your strengths? This will help you get past the thoughts that stand in your way and, who knows, it could be the shape of things to come.

Chapter Fourteen

A True Survivor

'Never, never, never give up.'

WINSTON CHURCHILL

One of the women who has had a positive impact on my life and a profound influence on my recovery is Professor Jane Plant, one of Britain's most distinguished scientists. Her lifestyle programme to reduce the risk of cancer has reached millions of women who have been touched by the disease. Jane was awarded, the Lord Lloyd Prize for her work in the field of science.

Having been given two months to live, she astounded all the experts when she experienced a complete remission of her cancer. She has remained cancer-free for over 18 years now. In her book *Your Life in Your Hands* she gives a first-hand account of her personal story about battling breast cancer. This nightmare is hard for any woman to endure once but Jane's cancer returned five times and grew progressively worse, eventually spreading to her lymph system.

The following paragraphs are Jane's and her husband Peter's account of her inspiring story.

Jane had a busy lifestyle – she was a career woman with a full-time job and three children to take care of. She had become ill-nourished because of what she read about food-industry recommendations, and she survived on what was marketed and advertised as health food and low-fat food. She ate large quantities of dairy food, skimmed-milk, organic yogurt, cottage cheese and dishes made of meat from dairy cows, which she washed down with milky tea. Jane told me about her lifestyle before her diagnosis.

> *Although I ate a lot of fruit and cereals, I had few salads and vegetables in my diet. I simply took high-dose vitamin C pills and multivitamin and mineral pills to ensure I covered any deficiencies.*

As we discussed her terrifying experience, she recounted the ordeal of being diagnosed with breast cancer five times.

> *I was first diagnosed in 1987 in October, and although I was free for five years, it came back another 4 times in 1993. I had all the orthodox treatments, a mastectomy, radiation, chemotherapy, my ovaries irradiated. Yet, despite the fact that I was seen by some of the UK's most eminent specialists, I have to admit I felt I was part of a machine. Once they realised I was a government scientist, they tolerated my questions and tried hard to answer and reassure me. In the end – and I literally mean the end – in order to gain control of my life, I relied on my scientific knowledge and experience.*

When she was told she had two months to live, if she was lucky, her response was why don't they end it now because she felt there was no point in going on. Then she heard Tom, her 11-year-old son, who is now a doctor asking, 'Where is Mummy?' At that moment, she knew she had to find a way to save her life. As we shared this emotional moment that any woman would find difficult to bear, Jane explained how she felt there had to be some sort of rational explanation.

> I suppose that's the scientist in me. Thankfully, that drove me to unearth the facts, some of which were known only to a handful of scientists at the time. I didn't choose to study breast cancer – it chose me. I did not pray for healing, I prayed that I would find out what I was doing wrong. I was desperate to live.

In spite of the devastating news, Jane decided to trust her scientific education and began to research the scientific facts about cancer. Her search for its causes led to the revelation that dairy products are the single most important factor causing breast cancer in Western women. Jane and her husband Peter began their desperate search to save her life. Peter, who is also a scientist, described to me how they had both worked in China as geologists for many years. As he shared the scientific facts they had learned about dairy products, I could tell he was just as passionate as Jane to get this message to the people.

> In all my time of working in China, I never saw one dairy cow and I worked in many different areas. The Chinese did not have a dairy industry, they did not eat dairy products. Our first clue to understanding what was promoting Jane's cancer came when I arrived back from a trip to China. Some colleagues gave me some huge herbal suppositories. My Chinese colleagues believed they were a cure for breast cancer. Despite the

devastating news, we both laughed because they looked like firework rockets. I remember Jane saying that it was no wonder that Chinese women avoided getting the disease if this was the treatment for breast cancer in China. Those words echoed in our minds. Why didn't Chinese women get breast cancer?

Jane and Peter began to brainstorm to see if they could find a link. When they looked at the maps they found breast cancer was virtually non-existent throughout the whole country. In fact, in rural China only 1 in 10,000 women were diagnosed with breast cancer each year, rather than the 1 in 9 lifetime risk in the West. Statistics of epidemiological maps of China had no reference of prostate cancer because the incidence of that particular cancer was so low. Even in industrialised Hong Kong, the rates were still low, only 34 women in every 10,000 were affected by breast cancer. Hiroshima and Nagasaki had similar rates and as both those cities had been attacked by nuclear bombs, you would expect to find some radiation-related cases in those cities.

'These statistics bring home the realisation that if a Western woman were to move to industrialised, irradiated Hiroshima, she would reduce her risk of contracting breast cancer by half,' Peter said in a convincing tone.

'In the back of my mind, I remember that the Chinese people had a slang name for breast cancer – 'rich woman's disease'. It seems to affect people that are in higher socio-economic groups, those who can afford to eat rich foods. It is quite disturbing to see how the rates in the West have risen over the past few years, the odds are high if you live in the West. Clearly the Chinese were doing something to protect themselves against cancer,' Jane continued.

This highlighted to them that there must be some lifestyle factor that was seriously increasing Western women's chance of contracting breast cancer. They wondered if its causes were genetic but the research showed that when Chinese or Japanese people move to the West, within one or two generations their rates of breast cancer approach the norms of the country they have moved to.

When they made the connection that Oriental women have very low rates of breast cancer, Peter and Jane began to wonder if dairy was a significant dietary component in the cause of the disease. They researched a number of scientific studies that pointed to the fact that the growth factors that are contained in dairy products help the production of the insulin-like growth factor-I (IGF-I), which is an aggressive promoter of cancer and abnormal cell growth.

Peter recalled only being given milk once when he had been in China – and that had been brought from a nearby city by some of his colleagues because they had heard that Western people liked it. He realised if they had to go to such lengths to get milk, then it could not be part of their diet. Jane recollected that traditional Chinese people never feed their babies dairy food, much less adults, and many of her Chinese friends were unable to tolerate milk.

After this bit of insight, they just used logic and scientific fact to come to the conclusion that dairy-product consumption is as much a risk factor for breast cancer (and perhaps prostate cancer), as smoking is for lung cancer. Jane believes that cow's milk is a perfect food for a rapidly growing baby calf, but it is not intended by nature for consumption by any species other than baby cows.

She is convinced that milk from dairy cows, is responsible for a share of Western health problems. The evidence is pretty compelling when we address the fact that the Chinese also have the lowest rates of osteoporosis in the world and yet consumed no dairy products.

As many of my readers suffer from arthritis, osteoporosis, congestion and are lactose intolerant, I did my own research. What I found lacking was scientific support for consuming foods that have adverse effects on the body. Epidemiological research suggests a correlation between milk consumption and at least two kinds of cancer, breast and prostate. The research shows that casein, a group of proteins found in milk, is a chemical carcinogen.

The first thing that strikes you about our habit of drinking milk is that we are drinking the milk of another animal. Is it unnatural for humans to drink milk from another species? Humans have not evolved to drink milk that contains bovine growth hormones. Moreover, cows are exposed to pesticides and antibiotics and are also milked when they are pregnant, which is a time when these animals have increased levels of oestrogens.

Large mammals such as elephants and silver back gorillas have huge muscle structures, yet they do not suffer with osteoporosis and they eat no dairy. Wild animals seem to have figured out the foods that nourish their bodies, of course animals use their natural instincts. What is it that has separated man from our natural instincts? Could it be the result of clever marketing?

Another fact that distinguishes us from other animals is that we are the only species to continue to drink milk after weaning. Is that because we are concerned that we will not get enough calcium and protein if we don't consume dairy products? The core of the dairy argument is that we will not get enough calcium to sustain strong bones if we don't consume dairy products. Yet, studies show that by consuming dairy products that minerals disappear from our bones, which weakens them and subjects them to arthritis and osteoporosis.

Head of the Physicians Committee for Responsible Medicine, Neal Barnard, says, 'It would be hard to imagine a worse vehicle for delivering calcium to the human body.'

Dr Colin Campbell, nutritional biochemist at Cornell University confirms:

> *Although milk's calcium and other nutrients do promote bone growth, other substances in dairy foods such as proteins and sodium actually leach some calcium from bone.*

It is lack of weight-bearing exercise that decreases bone density. Strength training strengthens bone.

As for any concerns about getting enough proteins, well babies do not suffer protein deficiencies on breast milk which contains small amounts of proteins (approximately 3 to 5 per cent), in fact they double and triple in size during a very short period. Dairy milk also causes the body to produce mucus, especially in the gastro-intestinal tract. This type of reaction in the body is produced when the immune system tries to clean animal proteins out of the body.

Jane's research has contributed to public understanding of the potential health hazards of drinking dairy milk. This led her into much controversy with the dairy industry and its advertisers. While promoting her book in the USA, she appeared on prime-time television. After her appearance, her scheduled engagements with other networks were cancelled without explanation. Jane is not daunted by the might of the dairy industry, she continues to work tirelessly to expose the risks of drinking milk. After years of scientific research, not one drop of milk has passed her lips.

It can of course be difficult to give up what we have become accustomed to for most of our lives – I know many of my own friends are absolutely addicted to cheese – but I doubt that we can continue to ignore the risk factors that these growth hormones pose to our health. While there are conflicting views about the consumption of these products there can be no disagreement that breast cancer has reached epidemic rates in many Western countries.

Jane raised her eyebrows as she explained that she had also discovered that the vast majority of the world's population are unable to digest the milk sugar, lactose.

'I wonder if nature is trying to tell us that we are eating the wrong food?' she said steadfastly.

When Jane eliminated all dairy products from her diet, she threw the milk down the sink and cheese in the bin. Within days, the lump in the lymph nodes in her neck had started to shrink, she tracked the tumour's progress with callipers (an instrument that she had used to measure fossils) as it began to regress, six weeks later she could not find it. She became very experienced at detecting cancerous tumours, she discovered all five of her cancers herself.

> *I check for lumps regularly – self-examination saved my life. I have a false boob now. Breast cancer changed me from being insecure and easily persuaded by authority into a stronger woman. My specialist was as overjoyed as I was. Of course when I first discussed my ideas with him, he was understandably sceptical.*

Jane has remained cancer free for 18 years. She wrote her touching book *Your Life in Your Hands,* and a follow up book *The Plant Programme* in order to help others gain insight into how they too could improve their chances of recovery. Her research and down-to-earth advice is a symbol of hope to those newly diagnosed. With the staggering increase of breast cancer in the West, she encourages women to take an active role in the prevention and treatment of their disease.

Having come to know Jane over the past few years, one of the most extraordinary things I have noticed about her is her incredible determination. She did not surrender, even though there is no doubt that she has been tested to her limits and has endured much pain and anguish, but her success was born of the dramas of her personal suffering. She vows that her lifestyle has saved her life. As she shared the lessons she learned on her personal journey, her advice to others searching for solutions is:

> *Find something you trust, stick with it and make sure it is not controlled by vested interests. It is changing your body chemistry*

by changing your diet and lifestyle that is the crucial thing to do.

Our conversation about her recovery was of more than just scientific facts, the depth of her relationship with Peter was no doubt a wonderful support to Jane throughout each of her diagnoses. Jane is a survivor in every sense of the word, her energy, knowledge and profound commitment to help others is evident. Her exacting standards and insistence on clarity and establishing facts means that she continues to be consulted on various matters of health. Her message is wonderful, uplifting news for every person who fears cancer. After her amazing survival this humble and compassionate woman's fame has grown through those who pass on her story. I hope I have portrayed Jane's simple message that even advanced breast cancer can be overcome because she has done it. She is living proof of what it means to have a *survivor's mindset*.

Further Reading

Antczak, S. & Antczak, G. (2001). *Cosmetics Unmasked.* Wellingborough: Thorsons.

Benson, H. & Epstein, M. D. (1975). 'The Placebo Effect: A Neglected Asset in the Care of Patients'. *Journal of the American Medical Association,* 232, pp. 1225–7.

Bernay-Roman, A. (2001). *Deep Feeling, Deep Healing.* London: Spectrum Press.

Binzel, P. E. (1994). *Alive and Well.* New York, NY: American Media.

Bohan, B. (2011). *The Choice.* Dublin: Gill & Macmillan.

Bohan, B. (2011). *The Choice: The Programme.* London: HarperThorsons.

Brazier, B. (2004). *Thrive.* Coquitlam, BC: Oceanside.

Brofman, M. (2003). *Anything Can Be Healed.* Forres, Scotland: Findhorn Press.

Burney, L. (2004). *Immunity Foods for Healthy Kids.* London: Duncan Baird.

Caldara, L. (2006). *180 Ways to Effectively Deal With Change.* Flower Mound, TX: Walk the Talk Company.

Campbell, C. & Campbell, T. (2005). *The China Study.* Dallas, TX: BenBella.

Capra, F. (1982). *The Turning Point.* New York, NY: Simon & Schuster.

Clements, B. (1998). *Living Foods for Optimum Health.* Rocklin, CA: Prima Health.

Colman, A. M. (2006). *Oxford Dictionary of Psychology* (2nd edition). Oxford: Oxford University Press.

Cotter, A. (1999). *From This Moment On.* New York, NY: Random House.

Daniel, R. (2003). *Eat to Beat Cancer.* Wellingborough: Thorsons.

Daniel, R. (2005). *The Cancer Directory.* Wellingborough: Thorsons.

Day, P. (1999). *Cancer: Why we're still Dying to Know the Truth.* Kent: Credence Publications.

Day, P. (2005). *The Little Book of Attitude.* Kent: Credence Publications.

de Bono, E. (2004). *How to have a Beautiful Mind.* London: Vermilion.

Dossey, L. (2006). *The Extra-Ordinary Healing Powers of Ordinary Things.* New York, NY: Harmony.

d'Raye, T. (2001). *What's the Big Deal About Water?.* Portland, OR: Awieca Inc.

Edgson, V. & Marber, I. (1999). *The Food Doctor.* London: Collins & Brown.

Epstein, G. (1989). *Healing Visualizations.* New York, NY: Bantam Books.

Erasmus, U. (1993). *Fats that Heal, Fats that Kill.* Burnaby, BC: Alive Books.

Gross, R. D. (2001). *The Science of Mind and Behaviour* (4th edition). London: Hodder & Stoughton.

Groves, B. (2001). *Fluoride: Drinking Ourselves to Death.* Dublin: Gill & Macmillan.

Gursche, S. (1997). *Encyclopaedia of Natural Healing.* Burnaby, BC: Alive Books.

Gursche, S. (2000). *Juicing – for the Health of it.* Burnaby, BC: Alive Books.

Hamilton, D. R. (2009). *It's the Thought that Counts.* Carlsbad, CA: Hay House.

Holford, P. (2007). *Optimum Nutrition for the Mind.* London: Piatkus.

Janov, A. (2007). *The Janov Solution.* Pittsburgh, PA: SterlingHouse Books.

Jordan, D. S. (1984). *The Philosophy of Despair.* Nashville, TN: W Publishing Company. This book was originally published in 1902 and is available to download as a free e-book from many websites.

Leggett, D. (1999). *Recipes for Self-Healing.* Totnes, Devon: Meridian Press.

Lipton, B. (2009). *The Biology of Belief.* Carlsbad, CA: Hay House.

Lono Kahuna Kupua A'o (1996). *Don't Drink the Water.* Pagosa Springs, CO: Kali Press.

McEoin, B. (2001). *Boost Your Immune System Naturally.* London: Carlton.

Maslow, A. (1971). *The Farther Reaches of Human Nature.* New York, NY: Viking.

Maslow, A. (1998). *Toward a Psychology of Being* (3rd edition). San Francisco, CA: Wiley Publishing.

Melcombe, L. (2000). *Health Hazards of White Sugar.* Burnaby, BC: Alive Books.

Mercola, Dr (2004). *Total Health.* www.mercola.com.

Montagu, A. (1986). Touching: The Human Significance of the Skin (3rd edition). New York, NY: Harper & Row.

Moran, V. (1985). *Compassion: The Ultimate Ethic.* Wellingborough: Thorsons.

O'Bannon, K. (2000). *Sprouts.* Burnaby, BC: Alive Books.

O'Regan-Caryle, B. (1993). *Spontaneous Remission.* Petalumas, CA: Hirshberg Institute of Noetic Sciences.

Pert, C. (1999). *Molecules of Emotion.* New York, NY: Scribner.

Plant, J. (2000). *Your Life in Your Hands.* London: Virgin.

Plant, J. & Tidey, G. (2001). *The Plant Programme.* London: Virgin.

Rotter J. (1966). 'Generalized expectancies of internal versus external control of reinforcements'. *Psychological Monographs,* 80.

Seligman, M. E. P. (1975). *Helplessness: On Depression, Development and Death.* San Francisco, CA: W.H. Freeman.

Servan-Schreiber, D. (2008). *A New Way of Life.* New York, NY: Viking.

Silva, J. & Goldman, B. (1990). *The Silva Mind Control Method*. London: Grafton Books.

Simonton, C. (1992). *Getting Well Again*. New York, NY: Bantam.

Steinman, D. & Epstein, S. S. (1995). *The Safe Shopper's Bible*. San Francisco, CA: Wiley Publishing.

Taubert, P. M. (2001) *Silent Killers – more than you paid for*. Murray Bridge, South Australia: Comp Safe Consultancy.

Thomas, P. (2001). *Cleaning Yourself to Death*. Dublin: Gill & Macmillan.

Tolle, E. (2005). *A New Earth*. New York, NY: Penguin.

Tusek D., Church, J. M. & Fazio, V. M. (1997). 'Guided Imagery as a Coping Strategy for Perioperative Patients'. *Aorn Journal*, Vol. 66(4), pp. 644–9.

Vale, J. (2002). *Slim 4 Life*. Wellingborough: Thorsons.

Vale, J. (2003). *The Juice Master's Ultimate Fast Food*. Wellingborough: Thorsons.

Vale, J. (2004). *Chocolate Busters*. Wellingborough: Thorsons, 2004.

Waitley, D. (1979). *The Psychology of Winning*. New York, NY: Berkeley Books.

Walker, N. (1995). *Water Can Undermine Your Health*. Prescott, AR: Norwalk Press.

Weil, A. (1995). *Spontaneous Healing*. London: Little Brown.

Wheater, C. (2001). *Juicing for Health*. Wellingborough: Thorsons.

Resources

To contact Bernadette for seminars, wellness programmes and information on supplements and health:

email: b@changesimply.com

or visit: www.changesimply.com

Resources in Ireland

Mind and Body Healing
7 Fair Street
Drogheda
County Louth

63 Park Street
Dundalk
County Louth

Blackcastle Centre
Navan
County Meath

LoCall 1890-252-567 (086-890-9541)
email: info@irishhypnosis.ie
www.irishhypnosis.ie

Healing Centre

Hippocrates Health Institute
1443 Palmdale Court
West Palm Beach
Florida 33411
telephone:00-1-561-471-8876
www.hippocrates.inst.com

Stockist of Juicer and Dehydrators

Naturalife Health Ltd
Rathnew
County Wicklow
telephone: 0404-62444
email: info@naturalife.ie
www.naturalife.ie

Reverse Osmosis Systems and Whole House Water Systems

Renewell Water Group
telephone: 042-9371940; 086-7335874
email: business@renewellwater.com; info@renewellwater.com
www.renewellwater.com

Wheatgrass, Fresh Sprouts and Organic Food Delivery Services

Living Green
Ballinclea
Donard
County Wicklow
telephone: 045-404683; 087-950-9598
email: info@livinggreen.ie
www.livinggreen.ie

The Happy Pear Living Foods
Leabeg Lower,
Newcastle,
County Wicklow
telephone: 086-101-4181
email: sprouts@livingfoods.ie
www.livingfoods.ie

Absolutely Organic
telephone: 01-460-0467
email: info@absolutelyorganic.ie

Safe Personal-Care Products

New Vistas Healthcare Ltd
7 Plassey Park
Limerick
telephone: 061-334455
fax: 061-331515
email: info@newvistashealthcare.com
www.newvistashealthcare.com

EO Ireland
62 Winter Garden
Pearse Street
Dublin 2
www.eoireland.com

Renaissance Products
Renaissance House
Church Street
Howth
County Dublin
telephone: 01-832-1412
email: reception@renaissanceproducts.com
www.renaissance-skincare.com

Resources in the United Kingdom

Stockist of Juicer and Dehydrators
Savant Distribution Ltd
Quarry House
Clayton Wood Close
Leeds, LS16 6QE
telephone: 08450-60-60-70
email: info@savant-health.com
www.savant-health.com

Reverse Osmosis Systems and Whole House Water Systems
Water Filter Man Ltd
89 Woodland Road
Wolverhampton
West Midlands, WV3 8AP
telephone: 0844 873 3148 (LoCall call rate);
00-44-1902-836688
email: info@waterfilterman.co.uk
www.waterfilterman.co.uk

Organic Food Delivery Services

The Fresh Food Company
telephone: 00-44-208-749-8778
www.freshfood.co.uk

Safe Personal-Care Products

Forever Natural UK
The Old Barrel Store
Brewery Courtyard
Drayman's Lane
Marlow
Buckinghamshire, SL7 2FF
telephone: 00-44-1628-891700
fax: 00-44-1628-891701

Useful websites

www.changesimply.com
www.voice.buz.org
www.irishlivingfood.com
www.cancerdecisions.com